Heal Your Gut

an A to Z guide
Healthy Bowel Healthy Body

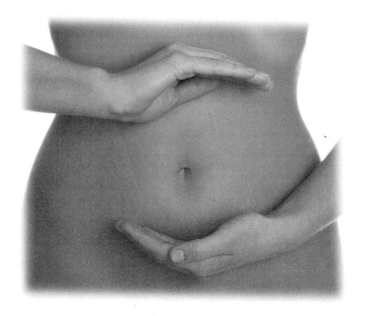

Sandra Cabot MD

Published by SCB International Inc.
2027 W Rose Garden Lane Phoenix, AZ 85027

Ph +1 623 334 3232

Website: www.liverdoctor.com
Website: www.sandracabot.com

© Sandra Cabot MD, 2017

ISBN 978-1-936609-21-5

HEA039010   HEALTH & FITNESS / Diseases / Gastrointestinal
HEA048000   HEALTH & FITNESS / Diet & Nutrition / General
HEA032000   HEALTH & FITNESS / Alternative Therapies

Contents

Contents

The Author

Sandra Cabot MD is a well known media doctor and author of 27 books on health, including the award winning Liver Cleansing Diet Book.

Dr Sandra Cabot is a consultant to the Women's Health Advisory Service, regularly appears on Australian TV shows and radio, and is a much sought after public speaker on the health issues of our time.

Sandra is sometimes known as the "Flying Doctor" as she frequently flies herself to many country towns to hold health seminars for women and increasingly also for men. These help to raise funds for local community services and women's refuges. Sandra has spent considerable time working in a large missionary hospital in the Himalayan foothills of India.

Sandra receives thousands of emails from people from all over the world who have read her books and are searching for holistic solutions to their health problems.

Her mailing address is ehelp@liverdoctor.com

Preface

Hippocrates the father of medicine said that all diseases begin in the gut. Well we have come a long way since Hippocrates, and have discovered that many diseases are genetic in origin; but it is still true today that if your digestive tract is unhealthy you will not be a healthy individual even if you have been lucky enough to inherit an excellent set of genes (genome). After nearly 40 years of practicing medicine I do believe that good health and longevity is dependent on the health of the digestive tract and liver.

The most basic necessity of life is to supply the body with good nutrition and water. The enjoyment of food is one of life's great pleasures and brings us together as human beings. But for many the enjoyment of food and the supply of nutrients essential to good health can be greatly impaired by disorders of the intestinal tract. You may eat a nutritious diet but if your liver, pancreas or intestines are not healthy you will not be able to benefit from the nutrients in healthy foods.

However the digestive tract is far more than a source of pleasure and nutrients, and over the last decade we have come to understand that the gut plays a crucial role in all aspects of our health. We have discovered links between the gut and mental health, diabetes, immune dysfunction, obesity and autism. The relationship between gut health and mental health is especially interesting as the gut has now become recognized as the second "brain". This is because the intestines produce the largest supply of neurotransmitters (biogenic amines) and indeed produce a lot more serotonin than the brain does. Serotonin is known as the "happy neurotransmitter" as it affects our mood, sleep and energy. The brain-gut connection is being researched and we know that the state of our gut has a huge effect on our mental health. If there is inflammation in the gut there can be inflammation in the brain and this can lead to mood disorders and disorders of the nervous system.

Our whole body is hugely affected by the microorganisms in our gut and this mass of bacteria is known as the microbiome. If the microbiome is unbalanced and unhealthy bacteria predominate, this will produce inflammation that causes widespread stress on all parts of our body. The human genome contains approximately 35,000 genes and the amount of genes in the microbiome is around one million genes; thus human genes are far less numerous than our bacterial genes.

This book will give you the vital principles for a healthy digestive system and the techniques to treat and reverse different types of intestinal and bowel problems. It also provides delicious liver and bowel healthy recipes for enjoyment and to heal your gut problem.

Chapter 1

What is the digestive system

The digestive tract is known as the alimentary canal and is a muscular tube around 10 meters (33 feet) long that starts at the mouth and ends at the anus.

Along the huge length of the digestive tract there are many things that can go wrong from bad breath to hemorrhoids.

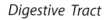

Digestive Tract

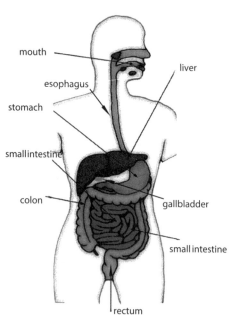

Digestion begins in the mouth, where food is chewed and mixed with saliva from the salivary glands. Saliva contains the enzyme amylase that begins to break down starches in the food. Food then travels down the esophagus by a muscular contraction called the peristaltic movement. Once the food reaches the stomach, the hormone gastrin is secreted which stimulates the secretion of hydrochloric acid, which enables more digestion of the food.

After being processed by the stomach the food is no longer in a solid state and is now a liquid called chyme. The chyme travels into the first part of the small intestine called the duodenum. In the duodenum the majority of food digestion occurs because multiple enzymes, released by the pancreas and bile from the bile duct are secreted. In the duodenum carbohydrates are broken down into simple sugars, the protein into amino acids, and the fats into glycerol and fatty acids. These substances are absorbed into the blood stream by cells lining the intestines. Substances that cannot be broken down or absorbed then pass to the large intestine (colon). In the colon the last of the water, ions, and salts are reabsorbed, and the remaining solid material, called feces, exits through the anus. Thus, the digestive tract is a passageway for food to be ingested transported, broken down, absorbed, and expelled.

Digestive Tract

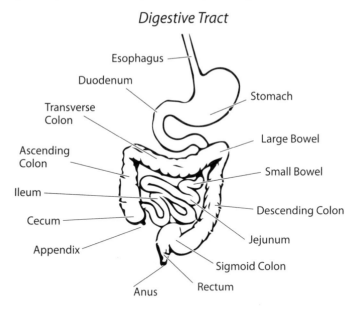

The term bowels is synonymous with the intestines or the gut. The small intestines are referred to as the small bowel. The small bowel has 3 parts. The part nearest the stomach is called the duodenum, the next part is the jejunum and the third part is the ileum, which connects with the large intestine. The large intestine is known as the colon.

Where the ileum joins the large bowel (at the cecal area of the colon), there is a valve called the ileo-cecal valve.

The Colon

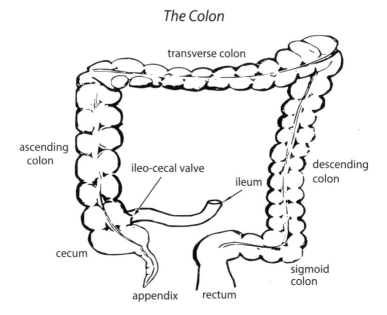

The ileo-cecal valve is designed to stop particles and feces from refluxing backwards into the ileum.

The ileum is a vitally important part of the small intestine because it is here that vitamin B 12 and the bile salts are absorbed. If the ileum becomes diseased, as in Crohn's disease, severe nutritional deficiencies can result leading to serious diseases.

The large intestines or large bowel are divided into the colon and the rectum. The first part of the colon has a sac like shape and is called the cecum, which is the site of attachment of the appendix. The colon has an upside down U shape, and goes from the ascending colon to the transverse colon to the descending colon, and finally the sigmoid colon, which joins the rectum. The main function of the colon is the absorption of water from the processed food residue that arrives after essential nutrients have been absorbed in the small intestine. The last part of the large bowel is the rectum, which is a reservoir for feces, which are stored until the urge to pass a bowel motion is felt. Problems can occur if the size of the colon becomes too large, or if it develops inflammation, spasm or pockets (diverticula) in its muscular walls. These are common problems in people who consume the typical Western diet.

Causes of Intestinal and Digestive Problems

• Liver problems such as sluggish liver function or fatty liver or liver disease.

• Gall bladder problems such as a non-functioning gallbladder or gallstones often cause nausea and indigestion after eating and/or discomfort over the right upper abdomen or pain referred to the right shoulder. Some people experience chronic indigestion and/or diarrhea after losing their gallbladder and treatment is available to help these problems. Supplements of ox bile and digestive enzymes can help to relieve these symptoms. For more information see my book titled How to Save Your Gallbladder and what to do if you have lost it.

• Some medications - non steroidal anti-inflammatory drugs, aspirin and/or high dose oral pain killers can cause ulcers and bleeding from the stomach and small intestines. Pain killers slow down the muscle contractions of the intestines often causing constipation. Antacid drugs which stop acid production in the stomach may reduce the digestion and absorption of nutrients from the intestines. These drugs reduce hydrochloric acid production by the stomach, and although sometimes needed for bad reflux, may have damaging side effects. Lack of hydrochloric acid production in the stomach increases the risk of intestinal infections with unfriendly bugs; this is because hydrochloric acid is needed to kill bacteria, parasites and fungi. Also, inadequate production of hydrochloric acid reduces the ability to digest protein foods and reduces the absorption of minerals such as calcium. This increases the risk of osteoporosis.

Antibiotic drugs can be damaging to the intestines. Antibiotic drugs kill not only the bad bacteria; they also kill off all the good bacteria, which are so essential for a healthy bowel and immune system. Antibiotic drugs can lead to an overgrowth of unfriendly opportunistic bacteria and fungi and this can lead to a leaky gut. The after effects on the gut of repeated or prolonged courses of antibiotics can take many months to recover from and the strategies in this book will speed up healing of the gut. Past chemotherapy and radiation therapy can damage the intestinal lining.

• Poor diet lacking in vegetables and fruits and consumption of processed foods, which contain preservatives, sugar, hydrogenated fats and chemical additives. A high intake of refined sugar and sugary foods is very detrimental to intestinal health and promotes fungal infections (such as candida) and unhealthy intestinal bacteria (dysbiosis).

• Food allergies and intolerances can cause irritable bowel syndrome. The most common food intolerances are to lactose (found in dairy products) and fructose (fruit sugar), fructans and other fructo-oligosaccharides (these are known as FODMAPs). If you are intolerant to these types of carbohydrates you will have excess bloating and a lot of flatulence and perhaps diarrhea. You will need to see a dietitian to follow what is known as a low FODMAP diet. "FODMAPs" stands for Fermentable-Oligo-Di and Mono-saccharides and Polyols. For more information see page 133. There is a lot of good information about FODMAPs on the Internet and yet many sufferers remain undiagnosed.

• Gluten intolerance can cause celiac disease; this is where the lining of the small bowel is so damaged that nutrients and fat cannot be absorbed. However gluten intolerance may not cause celiac disease but can still damage the intestines in other ways – this may cause symptoms of irritable bowel or constipation or leaky gut. Gluten intolerance can lead to bowel inflammation and can worsen the conditions of bowel polyps, ulcerative colitis and Crohn's disease. A good test to see if you are prone to gluten intolerance or celiac disease is a blood test, which checks your HLA DQ Genotype to see if you carry the genes associated with celiac disease. However the best test is to avoid gluten in your diet for 3 months and observe the difference in your bowel health. You can still have intestinal intolerance to gluten even if the Genotype test and celiac serology tests are negative.

• Lack of fluid intake, especially water, can lead to constipation and bowel toxicity. Indeed chronic dehydration is a very common cause of bowel and digestive problems. If you have bowel problems you need to drink plenty of healthy fluids such as water, herbal teas and vegetable juices. Try to drink 10 glasses of these types of fluids daily to rehydrate your whole body.

• Lack of digestive enzymes from the pancreas. The pancreas may be damaged from a build up of fat within it (fatty pancreas) or excess alcohol or sugar. This can be helped by taking digestive enzyme capsules at the beginning of meals. See page 22

• Autoimmune disease may attack the stomach lining causing inability to absorb vitamin B 12 from the small intestines and this can be detected by low blood vitamin B 12 levels. Autoimmune disease can also attack the small and large intestines causing Crohn's disease and ulcerative colitis

• Stress, anxiety and rushing your meals (as well as unpleasant people!) can cause indigestion and irritable bowel syndrome. It can really make a difference if you try and relax before you eat, slow down and chew your food thoroughly.

The most common bowel problems include:

• Sluggish contractions of the muscular walls of the stomach and intestines; this is called intestinal dysmobility or a lazy bowel; this usually results in constipation and bloating. This can be caused by diabetes, excess and prolonged use of laxative drugs, diseases of the nervous system and spinal misalignment with nerve impingement.

• Reflux of acid contents from the stomach which flows back into the esophagus causing heartburn.

• Inflammation of the lining of the stomach known as gastritis or inflammation of the duodenum; this can lead to peptic ulcers which may bleed or rupture.

• An excessively long or redundant bowel which is too large; this affects around one in ten persons (10% of the population). A redundant bowel causes chronic constipation and bloating. This is sometimes called a "megacolon." People who have inherited such a long enlarged bowel usually complain of constipation from a young age. These people may not have a bowel action for many days unless they take large doses of laxatives.

• Pockets or diverticula in the wall of the colon – this is known as diverticulosis. These pockets often trap tiny pieces of food and can become inflamed and infected.

• Unhealthy types of parasites and fungi (such as candida and other yeasts, tape worms, round worms, amoeba, and blastocysts etc.) may inhabit the intestines. Pathogenic bacteria such as Helicobacter Pylori, E-coli and Clostridium difficile etc. may reside in the stomach and/or small and large bowel - this condition of unhealthy micro-organisms in the intestines is common and is called dysbiosis.

• An inflamed or thin lining (mucous membranes) of the intestines. This causes excess permeability of the bowel lining - this is known as leaky gut. If the inflammation becomes very severe, ulceration of the lining of the bowel may occur. A leaky gut increases the risk of immune dysfunction such as inflammation, food sensitivities and allergies.

• A prolapsed bowel, which hangs down too low in the abdominal and pelvic cavities. This occurs because of weakening in the connective tissues which support the bowel and is worsened by chronic constipation and prolonged straining during a bowel action. Weakness of the pelvic floor from repeated childbirth or difficult childbirth will worsen a bowel prolapse and may cause constipation or fecal incontinence. Weakness of the abdominal muscles can also contribute to bowel prolapse and regular exercise such as pelvic floor exercises, Yoga and/or Pilates can help a lot.

Chapter 2

Strategies to help all types of Bowel Disorders

Improve Dietary Habits

Increase your intake of water. One of the most important and yet often overlooked strategies to improve bowel function for all people, is to drink more pure WATER. I cannot tell you how many people I have seen over the years with bowel problems who are chronically dehydrated. This causes the bowel contents to harden and stagnate, which can lead to overgrowth of bad bacteria and also increase inflammation of the bowel lining. I recommend at least 2 liters of suitable liquid daily (pure water, tea, and vegetable juices).

Increase your intake of fiber. Many people lack fiber because they eat refined sugars and carbohydrates, and too much processed food. Without fiber, the contents of the bowel will stagnate, which can lead to inflammation from excessive toxin formation. Lack of fiber will also force the bowel muscles to contract too strongly in an effort to move the feces along to the rectum to stimulate a bowel movement. These excessive contractions will increase the pressure inside the bowel, which leads to spastic colon and the formation of pockets in the bowel wall (diverticula). See diagram on page 59

Avoid excess alcohol as this can cause inflammation of the bowel wall and in some people alcohol causes a form of colitis.

Increase your intake of raw food. Forty percent of the diet should consist of RAW vegetables, fruits, nuts and seeds. In severe cases of candida it may be necessary to greatly reduce the amount of fruits and increase the intake of vegetables.

Raw foods contain active enzymes, natural antibiotics and active vitamins that improve digestion, fight unfriendly microorganisms and reduce inflammation of the bowel wall. We have plenty of yummy salad recipes in this book to keep you entertained. If you find it hard to digest raw fruits and vegetables invest in a high powered blender or food processor such as a Vitamix or Thermomix to produce raw delicious and easily digested recipes.

You can also start to eat some fermented foods to boost your gut population of friendly microorganisms and this can have enormous digestive and immune benefits – see page 254

For some it can be very hard to change old dietary habits and a new perspective may be needed. This was the case for Eric, a 52 year old bachelor who came to see me complaining of excessive weight gain, abdominal bloating, fatigue, sore joints and indigestion. He had been fully investigated and the only problem found was a fatty liver. He was a typical bachelor and that, combined with his high powered career of accounting, left him no spare time to follow a complicated dietary regime. He felt so unwell that he knew he had to change but the task was overwhelming to him. He lived on take away convenience and fast foods high in fat and sugar and did not go shopping.

With a mammoth effort Eric started to visit green grocers, butchers and super markets to source the foods that his liver needed to repair itself. After 8 weeks he returned and was happy to report that he felt much better and was losing weight easily. He had increased his energy levels and his mind was much sharper. He did however complain that the busy time of the year was approaching and that he could not see himself finding the time to continue shopping and preparing food. I suggested that he hire a domesticated woman who could shop for him and come to his home 2 days a week and prepare his meals, which could be refrigerated and stored hygienically. At first he complained that this would be expensive, however after we worked out the cost of continually eating out, he could see that he would actually save money and precious time. He would be able to pack a lunch to take to work from the food that the cook had left for him. This way he would have control over what he ate and be able to enjoy home cooked meals. I am happy to say that this worked out very well for him and he is continuing to improve and lose weight.

Improve Your Digestion and Absorption of Nutrients from Food

Some simple but often overlooked tips are –

- Chew food thoroughly

- Have teeth and jaw problems checked out early

- Do not eat very much if you are angry or stressed

- Do not over eat

- Drink only small amounts of liquids with meals because fluids will dilute the gastric juices needed for digestion.

Stomach acid

The lining of the stomach produces pepsin and rennin and hydrochloric acid, which provides the correct acidity for the digestive enzymes.

Deficiency of stomach hydrochloric acid is common in those over 60 years of age, and can lead to weakened digestion and multiple nutritional deficiencies, especially a deficiency of vitamin B 12. In such cases it is desirable to increase stomach acidity during meals, and this can be done with tablets of Betaine Hydrochloride. The usual dose is between 200 to 500 mg of Betaine Hydrochloride taken in the middle of a meal. Once dissolved in the stomach, Betaine Hydrochloride yields 25% of its weight as hydrochloric acid. Another tablet to increase hydrochloric acid is glutamic acid hydrochloride, which is slightly less potent and requires a dose of 600 to 1800 mg during meals.

Another useful technique to increase stomach acidity during a meal is to sip a glass of water containing 2 to 3 tablespoons of good quality organic apple cider vinegar with the juice of half a lemon or lime added. Some people find that this practice really improves their digestion and reduces flatulence and abdominal bloating.

Those with a severe deficiency of stomach hydrochloric acid, (known as achlorhydria), may have an increased risk of stomach cancer and for this reason antioxidants such as vitamin C, E and selenium should be part of the daily supplementation program. Tests are available to test for stomach acid production – see page 269

Digestive Enzymes

If you find that you feel uncomfortable after eating a meal it is most worthwhile to try a supplement containing digestive enzymes. The pancreas produces digestive enzymes without which it is impossible to breakdown proteins, fats and carbohydrates. It is not uncommon for a slight to moderate deficiency of these pancreatic enzymes to occur, especially in those over 60 years of age. Lack of these enzymes will result in poor breakdown of proteins, fats and carbohydrates, leaving only partially digested food to pass through the bowel. This reduces absorption of vital nutrients and malnutrition of some degree will result. Furthermore partially digested proteins will be absorbed from the gut, which will overload the liver and may cause allergies.

The most efficient way to take the full complement of digestive enzymes is in the form of some type of whole pancreas preparation, which comes from animal sources. Such a suitable preparation is called Pancreatin and the dosage is 2 - 4 grams with each meal. If you do not like the thought of taking animal pancreas or you are a vegan, you may want to try a digestive preparation which contains enzymes from plants or the fungus aspergillus niger. For maximum effectiveness the enzyme supplement you choose should contain all of the major enzyme groups namely- amylase, lipase and protease. Keep your enzyme supplements in a cool dry place to ensure potency. Enzymes are available in capsule, powder and liquid forms

As we grow older the ability of the body to produce enzymes diminishes, and enzyme supplements can make a huge improvement to the digestive and nutritional health of persons over 50 years of age.

The body can also obtain enzymes from ingested food. Unfortunately food enzymes are extremely sensitive to heat, and even low to moderate heat destroys most of the enzymes in foods. This is one of the reasons I encourage people to eat more raw salads and fruits, as their active enzymes will improve your digestion. Foods that are high in enzymes are pineapples, apples, papaya, avocados, mangos and bananas. Sprouts are a potent source of digestive enzymes. Enzymes extracted from papaya and pineapples are available in tablet form and are called papain and bromelain respectively. Although they are proteolytic enzymes and can help with the digestion of proteins, they are not as powerful as a whole pancreatic supplement. There is an excellent digestive capsule called Super Digestive Enzymes Plus, which combine pancreas extract with Betaine hydrochloride and ox bile. These are particularly good if you experience digestive problems after losing your gallbladder. You may also need capsules of ox-bile as well as the digestive enzymes if you have lost your gallbladder or have liver disease. See www.liverdoctor.com

Microorganisms in your Bowel

Your bowels may be harboring excessive populations of unfriendly microorganisms such as fungi (most commonly yeasts such as candida albicans), bacteria, viruses and parasites. The term parasite is used to describe a great variety of creatures that vary in complexity from single celled organisms, all the way up to worms that may be several inches or longer. Common disease causing parasites are Giardia lambia, Entamoeba histolytica and Cryptosporidium, which can be difficult to detect with routine stool analysis and cultures. When a stool specimen is examined in the path laboratory for parasites, many of the yeasts that are seen are already dead. Stool cultures therefore often fail to reveal the presence of fungi even when the gut is heavily infected. Some laboratories will examine repeated fresh stool specimens obtained after inducing mild diarrhea with laxatives and this will increase the chances of detection. The specialized tests known as a "Complete Diagnostic Stool Analysis" (CDSA) can increase chances of detection – see page 263.

It can be difficult to eradicate intestinal parasites completely and many sufferers find that they keep on recurring. I have found that a medication called Niclosamide (brand name Yomesan) is the most effective drug against tape worm. Niclosamide belongs to the family of medicines called anthelmintics, which are medicines used in the treatment of worm infections. Niclosamide is used to treat broad or fish tapeworm, dwarf tapeworm, and beef tapeworm infections. Niclosamide may also be used for other tapeworm infections as determined by your doctor. It will not work for other types of worm infections (for example, pin worms or roundworms). A drastic saline purge (e.g. sodium sulphate, magnesium sulphate), given two hours after the Yomesan dose should ensure a rapid and complete expulsion of the worms. Without purging, the parasite is excreted in pieces during the next few days. Unfortunately this remedy is no longer marketed in Australia, however for those who have chronic problems with intestinal worms, you can contact the manufacturing company which is Bayer Australia. They may be able to help you.

A natural anti-parasite remedy that can sometimes be quite helpful is called Intestinal Para-Clean. See www.liverdoctor.com

Each capsule of Intestinal Para-Clean contains -

- Wormwood flower and leaf (Artemisia absinthium)100mg

- Black Walnut Green Hull (Juglaris nigra) 100mg

- Cloves (Syzygium aromaticum) 100mg

- Garlic (deodorized from Alium sativum) 50mg

- Butternut root bark (juglaris cinerea) 50mg

- Buckthorn bark (Rhamnus frangula) 50mg

- Pau D'Arco (Trabebuia heptaphylla Bark) 50mg

The Recommended Dose is to take one to two capsules, up to three times daily, just before food.

There is also a capsule formula available containing a combination of philodendron, oregano, thyme and clove essential oils, which can be prescribed by doctors and naturopaths – it is called BactoClear.

Anti-parasitic remedies are often more effective if they are followed by a purge, during which many dead parasites will be expelled in the feces. To achieve the required laxative effect you can take 2 to 3 teaspoons of Epsom salts with four glasses of water or fruit juice, two hours after finishing the anti- parasitic medication.

To reduce bowel infections with unfriendly bacteria, parasites and yeasts:

• Avoid refined sugars and carbohydrates, as they are the fuel for unhealthy microorganisms .

• Avoid preserved foods, especially preserved meats (pizza meats, corned beef, ham, devon, bacon, sausage, smoked meats and smoked fish etc)

• Avoid moldy foods such as old peanuts, green potatoes and dried fruits that are moldy or bitter.

• Avoid the long term or frequent use of antibiotic, anti-inflammatory and steroid drugs if possible.

• Eat plentiful fiber in the form of raw vegetables and fruits, whole grains (unless you are gluten intolerant), ground seeds, legumes (especially lentils) and raw or lightly cooked sweet corn. This will have a "broom effect" and sweep the walls of the colon removing layers of encrusted and hardened feces, which harbor unfriendly microorganisms. Use a gluten free fiber powder regularly, such as FiberTone to cleanse the colon.

• Follow practices of good hygiene such as sterilization of kitchen towels and washers and frequent hand washing. You can use a microwave oven to sterilize wet towels.

• Use natural antibiotics to reduce intestinal yeasts, bacteria and parasites. Natural antibiotic foods, herbs and condiments include cabbage juice, raw or fermented garlic, onions, leeks, radishes, fenugreek, ginger, chili, lemon juice, organic apple cider vinegar, turmeric, mustard and rosemary.

Garlic is able to kill bacteria, parasites and yeasts. Raw garlic cloves can be grated, chopped very finely, or pressed in a garlic press, and then mixed well throughout your cooked food and salads. It tastes nicer with some cold pressed olive oil and apple cider vinegar. Onions and leeks also have valuable antibiotic effects in the bowel, and if you cannot tolerate garlic you may find that these things work well for you.

Some naturopaths recommend tea or powder from Pau d'arco bark to fight yeast infections, while others recommend the 8-carbon fatty acid called Caprylic acid which is safe and may help in mild cases.

Typical herbs used to destroy and expel worms from the body are black walnut hulls, chaparral, cloves, liquorice, gentian and wormwood. All these herbs are combined together in Intestinal Para-Clean Capsules.

Take probiotic supplements and use plain Greek style sugar free yogurt to maintain ecological balance in the gut. They are particularly good after antibiotic therapy.

Those who are frequent international travelers are more at risk from infections such as hepatitis A and B and gut infections, and although vaccinations against many of these things are available today, it is still wise to protect your liver and immune system so that they can cope with this increased challenge. Practice good hygiene with frequent hand washing. Peel or slice the skin off from the fruit before eating and avoid raw salads, unless you are in a 5 star hotel! Make sure your food is well cooked. Drink only bottled water (carbonated is safer) or boiled water. You can add several drops of iodine and colloidal silver to your drinking water to reduce bacterial infections.

Probiotics

The word probiotic literally means to promote life. The term is now used to describe living microorganisms in the intestines that have positive health effects on an individual. The most well known probiotics are acidophilus and bifidus, but there are many others. An adult has approximately three kilograms of bacteria inside their intestines. We have far more bacterial cells inside and on the outside of our body than we have human cells. This may sound alarming but these bacteria are critical for our good health, and they are particularly important for healthy immune function. The vast amount of genetic material (DNA) in our body comes from the micro-organisms living inside our body and not from our own human cells.

Colonization of the intestines with bacteria begins at birth. While the fetus is inside its mother's uterus it is in a sterile environment. During labor, the infant is exposed to the mother's beneficial bacteria in the vagina. Babies that are born via cesarean section miss out on receiving a dose of good bacteria and this may increase their risk of developing immune system and digestive disorders. It is important to give these children a good probiotic supplement.

There are around 500 different species of bacteria in the intestines and new species are continually being discovered. The types of bacteria in your intestines, and their quantities, have a profound effect on your health. Good bacteria are anti-inflammatory, whereas bad bacteria secrete highly inflammatory substances into the gut. Having high levels of bad gut bacteria puts an enormous strain on your immune system and hugely increases the amount of inflammation and tissue destruction occurring in your body.

Dysbiosis is the term used to describe a bad balance of bugs in your gut (too many unhealthy bacteria and not enough good bacteria).

Factors that increase levels of pathological (unhealthy disease causing) bacteria in the gut include:

- Stress

- Poor dietary choices – especially excess sugar or alcohol consumption

- Food intolerances and food allergies

- Gastrointestinal infections from contaminated foods and water

- Medications – especially antibiotics, steroids, anti-inflammatory drugs and antacid drugs

A good probiotic supplement will help to correct the imbalance of bacteria in your intestines and will do wonders to reduce inflammation and help your immune system. It will also help to heal a leaky gut (excessively permeable intestinal lining). Eating yogurt is helpful but it must be unflavored and sugar free and still is not the most effective way to take a probiotic. In order to get the correct quantity and strains of bacteria, you will need to take a probiotic supplement. FloraTone-10 is a proprietary blend containing 10 clinically validated strains of bacteria containing 25 billion units of beneficial probiotics per serve.

FloraTone-10 capsules contain the following strains of healthy bacteria:

B.Longum, L. Rhamnosus, L. Paracasei, L. Acidophilus, B. Lactis, L. Casei, L. Plantarum, L. Salivarius, B. Breve, S. Thermophilus.

Another excellent way to increase the healthy bacteria in your intestines is to regularly consume fermented foods, which you can make at home or purchase – see page 254

Benefits of probiotics include:

• Digesting certain types of fiber, starches and sugars. The friendly bacteria in your digestive tract convert these substances into a source of energy and various acids which help to keep the bowel walls healthy. Food for good bacteria is called a prebiotic. Prebiotics are predominantly the indigestible fiber in certain vegetables and fruit. Jerusalem artichoke is a particularly rich source of prebiotics. This vegetable is in season during winter. Eating it will greatly increase the levels of good bugs in your bowel.

• Producing vitamins and eliminating toxins. Probiotics manufacture some vitamin K and improve your ability to absorb minerals. They also aid in the metabolism and the breakdown of toxins. This is beneficial because it means your liver will have to do less work breaking down toxic substances. Good bacteria produce short chain fatty acids, which are associated with lower levels of allergies and inflammation.

• Keeping bad bacteria under control. The helpful bacteria produce a substance that kills harmful microbes. It is literally a competition for space inside your digestive tract; the more good bacteria you have, the less room will be available for bad bacteria.

• Improving the integrity of the gut lining. Leaky gut syndrome, or an excessively permeable intestinal lining, is an extremely common condition and is often present in individuals with allergies and autoimmune disease. Good bowel bacteria help to repair and nourish the cells lining your gut and increase the integrity of the gut lining. This is important as it reduces the amount of toxins that get absorbed from the gut into the bloodstream.

• Preventing allergies. Good bacteria teach your immune system to distinguish between disease causing microbes and non-harmful antigens (such as foods), and to respond appropriately. This helps to prevent your immune system from over reacting to harmless substances such as proteins, thereby reducing your risk of allergies.

An enormous amount of research has shown that improving the composition of bacteria in your bowel greatly reduces your risk of eczema, asthma, hay fever, sinusitis and other allergic conditions.

• Help to support regular bowel motions and reduce the incidence of constipation.

• Supporting the immune cells inside your digestive tract. Approximately 70 to 80 percent of the immune cells inside your body are in your digestive tract. Good bacteria play a crucial role in the operation of the immune system and also help your immune cells to produce antibodies against disease causing microbes. Probiotics are beneficial for T regulatory cells, which are white blood cells that regulate the immune system and prevent excessive inflammation.

• Reduce the risk of vaginal infections. The composition of flora in your bowel directly determines the composition of your vaginal flora. Probiotics reduce the risk of bacterial infections in the vagina (bacterial vaginosis).

• Help to support a healthy body weight. It has recently been discovered that having high levels of good bacteria in your intestines makes it easier to lose weight and keep it off, whereas bad gut bacteria increases your risk of Syndrome X and type 2 diabetes.

Natural Remedies to help the Bowels

Aloe Vera

Aloe Vera juice can soothe the lining of the stomach and intestines and is useful for those with acid reflux, and stomach and duodenal ulcers. It is alkalinizing and can reduce the symptoms of excess stomach acid and reflux of stomach acid. Aloe Vera can be drunk as often as needed and is safe and harmless, unless of course, you are allergic to it. Do not take Aloe Vera juice with meals, as you need the stomach contents to be acidic to properly digest food. Take the Aloe Vera in between meals or if you have an acid reflux attack.

Grow some aloe vera plants in your garden and you will have a fresh supply. To learn how to grow and make your own aloe vera juice see appendix page 262

Antacids

Antacid medications are often used by those with excess gastric acidity and/or reflux. Avoid the long-term use of antacids containing aluminium. Some simple and harmless antacids are sodium and potassium bicarbonate, magnesium carbonate, magnesium hydroxide and calcium carbonate. A brand worth mentioning, that is free of aluminium, is Andrew's Tums.

Alfalfa juice or alfalfa tablets are alkaline and can soothe gastritis and/or reflux.

Fiber

A fiber powder called "FiberTone" is most helpful if you suffer with constipation. It is especially useful if your constipation is associated with irritable bowel syndrome, gluten intolerance, bowel pockets, colonic spasm or loss of the gallbladder. FiberTone contains psyllium husk, the amino acids Taurine and Glycine and the excellent liver herbs St Mary's Thistle and Dandelion root.

Herbs

The herbs golden seal, marshmallow, meadowsweet, liquorice, chamomile, peppermint, fennel and arrowroot can reduce intestinal colic and mild bowel inflammations. Digestive herbs such as dandelion, fennel, dill, aniseed, parsley, ginger and catnip can reduce burping and flatulence. Slippery elm powder can reduce acidity and reflux and soothes an irritable bowel. Slippery elm can be taken as a powder, capsules or tablets.

Condiments that reduce flatulence include caraway, cardamom, coriander, cumin, cloves, ginger and turmeric. Turmeric is a liver tonic and the usual dose is 1 - 2 tsp of the powder daily used to flavor food or mixed in juices. Turmeric is also a large component of curry powder.

Apple Cider Vinegar

Apple Cider Vinegar can help those with weak digestion due to low stomach acid production during meals. Drink or sip one to two tablespoons of apple cider vinegar diluted with an equal amount of water during meals. Choose an organic type which will be cloudy in appearance due to its probiotic content. It is also helpful for reducing bad bacteria in the gut.

Glutamine

Glutamine is an amino acid which provides fuel for the cells lining the intestines, and without it these cells waste away. Glutamine helps to protect and maintain the lining of the gastrointestinal tract (known as the mucosa). Normal metabolic and immune function of the intestines is dependent upon adequate amounts of glutamine.

Glutamine can be very beneficial in reducing the following:

- Leaky gut
- Autoimmune diseases of the intestines such as Ulcerative Colitis and Crohn's disease
- Gastritis
- Reflux
- Peptic ulcers

In critically ill patients, glutamine inhibits muscle wasting. Many people with cancer have abnormally low levels of glutamine in their body. Glutamine protects the liver during toxic chemotherapy, during paracetamol (acetaminophen) toxicity, and following a severe inflammatory injury to the liver. Glutamine is used to protect the lining of the gut from damage caused by chemotherapy or radiation. Glutamine may increase the effectiveness and reduce the side effects of chemotherapy treatments in cancer patients. If you are being treated for cancer, check with your doctor before using it.

In the advanced stages of AIDS (caused by infection with the human immunodeficiency virus (HIV)), patients often experience severe glutamine deficiency resulting in muscle loss. Glutamine combined with antioxidants may help people with AIDS to gain weight.

Glutamine, usually in the form of L-glutamine, is available by itself in powder, capsule or tablet form. The powder form allows higher doses to be used and quicker absorption. Take glutamine with cold or room temperature foods or liquids. It should not be added to hot beverages because heat destroys glutamine.

Children 8 years and younger: Do not give glutamine to a child unless your doctor recommends it.

Children 8 - 16 years: Doses of 500 - 1000 mg, 1 - 3 times daily, are generally considered safe.

Adults: Doses of 2500 to 5000mg, 1 - 2 times daily, are generally considered helpful.

Higher doses may be prescribed by a health care provider. Some people will benefit from much lower doses, of around 1000mg daily.

Healthy people do not need to supplement with glutamine. People with poor digestion, or those on long term antacid drugs, may not absorb amino acids efficiently and should benefit from glutamine. The typical dietary intake of L-glutamine is 5 to 10 grams daily. Supplemental dosages of glutamine range from 5 to 15 grams daily, divided into several separate doses.

Glutamine can be taken in water, juices or unsweetened milks, but not in hot beverages because heat destroys this amino acid. Glutamine supplements should also be kept in a dry location.

People with kidney disease or Reye syndrome (a rare, sometimes fatal disease of childhood that is generally associated with aspirin use) should not take glutamine.

A Case History of Bowel Parasites

by Trixi Whitmore

In 1994 I was diagnosed with "blastocystis homminis" found in a stool test and listed as "unknown pathogen" by the testing laboratory. My subsequent research discovered it to be a "protozoa". It is very widespread in the population and produces symptoms of bloating, flatulence and at times very explosive, smelly loose motions. At first these symptoms were spasmodic, but after a time they seemed to be present most of the time. Although I did not feel ill, I felt extra tired and just not "right"! The doctor did not offer or suggest any treatment. A subsequent visit to a specialist revealed that there was a severe outbreak in a country town and he was looking for a cure.

About this time my son suddenly developed symptoms which baffled the doctor. He had been away in Tasmania camping. The symptoms were terrifying and life-threatening. They began with acid indigestion, fatigue and constipation which became worse and worse each day. Antacid preparations were useless. He could eat less and less, had severe rumbling and grumbling in the tummy and the food and drink just seemed to stop at the navel level and took ages to digest. He went into a drugged-like sleep from which it was difficult to wake, and his hands and feet became swollen and very white. His face was ashen. After two weeks he had lost 14 kilograms (30 pounds) and finally when water would not pass through him, he was taken to hospital. Unfortunately it was the weekend and apart from an X ray he had no treatment. However the previous day he had seen a specialist who had prescribed Fasigyn, as he thought it could be an infection with the parasite giardia. The Fasigyn caused him agony, as it burnt from the throat down, but eventually after 30 hours, it must have trickled into his intestines as the "blockage" cleared.

After taking Slippery Elm to put a lining back onto his stomach, he started eating again, but after three days the symptoms recurred. Flagyl was then prescribed for one week and this brought things back to some kind of normality. However, he had become lactose intolerant and constipated, and had to be careful with food which was difficult to digest. This was a young man who had never had food allergies or bowel irregularities in his whole life.

Over the next 15 months the "bug" kept recurring about every six weeks. The Flagyl became useless. I kept trying different worm/parasite medicines for him, both herbal and allopathic, some of which worked for a short time, but the "bug" very quickly became immune to the remedy. Over this period I read everything I could about parasites, which I feel are far more prevalent in our country than are recognized! My son consulted various doctors and specialists who did not seem to realize the seriousness of the situation. "Irritable bowel syndrome" was the label! Unfortunately various tests were negative, but no-one stipulated that the most effective stool sample is a PURGED sample.

You might wonder why I have recounted the experience of my son? After 15 months I suddenly developed the same symptoms. (I suspect I may have picked it up while cleaning his toilet). My son had another relapse at the same time. After a week of terrible symptoms, when I had lost 6 kilograms (13 pounds), much searching discovered a herbal tapeworm remedy called Rascal, based on chili. This reversed the situation and our digestion started working again, but alas after three weeks it was ineffective. Further searching found a medicine called Yomesan (which unfortunately Bayer have removed from the Australian market). Yomesan is a tapeworm medicine and it worked and saved us from a fate worse than death, and has worked more than once. Yomesan treatment is followed by a purge with Epsom salts, which cleans out the dead worms.

Because I could not seem to get my digestion or bowels to return to normal, nor to get rid of the parasite problem, I finally consulted with a doctor who understood parasite problems. He sent my stool samples to The Great Smokies Laboratories in the USA for a test known as a CDSA (see page 263). These tests are now available in Australia at Health Scope, Nutripath and Analytical Reference Laboratories.

Great Smokies Lab found the parasites called Blastocystis Homminis and Dientamoeba Fragilis (which can be hosted by thread worms). They also discovered dysbiosis (unhealthy bacteria in the gut), rated at 12 on a scale of 1-10. Such was the health of my gut!

A long period of convalescence has now taken place with intermittent doses of Yomesan and other remedies, and I hope that both my son and I are beating the problem. All along I suspected that my son had something "different" - a very virulent "bug" which behaved in a different way to anything in the parasite literature, but responded to parasite medication. (I must thank Bayer for supplying me with such useful information on various parasites.)

After so many negative stool tests, I decided to start looking myself for evidence of worms. The ideal time was after dosing with Yomesan followed by Epsom salts. Persistence paid off, for I found some "interesting items," in my stool, which I took to a naturopath/biochemist. One of the "interesting items" I found was a definite worm, 6mm long, with a heart shaped tail. I photographed it, made a sketch of same, and took it to Newcastle University for identification. See diagram below. Also I sent the sketch and particulars to Dr. Leo Galland (world expert on parasites) and The Great Smokies Laboratories. So far no one can identify it! Maybe it is a new species of roundworm? Interestingly two new roundworms have recently been identified, one in Victoria in the muscle tissue of a fireman who was seriously ill, and another named crypto strongulus pulmoni in the sputum of chronic fatigue patients in the USA.

I now seem to be on the road to recovery with no evidence of blastocystis homminis in recent tests, but I do not know just what cured the blastocystis. Maybe it was the lemon juice and water first thing in the morning. However the dysbiosis was still a problem until a month ago, when I tried Olive Leaf Extract. This has had a remarkable effect. The bloating, wind and abnormal motions stopped and for the first time in years everything returned to normal. Heaven! Anyone diagnosed with "irritable bowel syndrome" or parasites should try it.

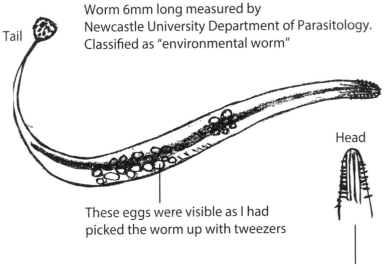

Tail

Worm 6mm long measured by
Newcastle University Department of Parasitology.
Classified as "environmental worm"

Head

These eggs were visible as I had
picked the worm up with tweezers

This was the pattern on the head of the worm

Chapter 3

Bowel Problems

Excess Intestinal Gas

Problems with excess intestinal gas and its transit through the gut are very common. Many people refer to it as excess wind inside them.

It is amazing to learn that around 25 liters of gas is produced inside the intestines every 24 hours!

So little wonder that abdominal bloating, belching (burping) and flatulence (farting) are so common.

Thankfully most of the gas produced is re-absorbed from the gut and the average amount of gas expelled daily from an adult is 1.5 to 3 liters. A lot of this gas expulsion occurs when you have a bowel action.

The gases produced in the intestines include hydrogen, hydrogen sulphide, oxygen, carbon dioxide, nitrogen, and methane – what a cocktail !

The passage of air from the anus is known as flatus and is often a noisy and smelly experience. The average person passes 2400mls (2.4 liters) of gas per day in portions of 30 to 120mls. The gases responsible for the strong odor are high in sulfur and are hydrogen sulphide, methanethiol, and dimethylsulphide. Thus eating healthy foods high in sulfur such as onions, garlic, eggs and cruciferous vegetables can increase this. Still it is better to be healthy as our liver and immune system need a lot of the mineral sulfur.

What can cause excess belching?

- Diseases of the esophagus such as reflux or inflammation

- Not chewing your food and rushing eating

- Lack of stomach acid can occur in people on antacid drugs

- Paralysis of the stomach muscles (known as gastroparesis)

- Disturbed motility of the muscles in the esophagus and/or stomach

- Inflammation of the stomach (gastritis) – see page 77

- Infections of the stomach with helicobacter pylori – see page 71

What can cause excess bloating?

- Eating too large a meal or rushing a meal

- Food intolerances – especially to dairy, gluten or foods high in FODMAPs – see page 133

- Dysfunction of the nerves to the muscles in the gut – this can occur due to stress, diabetes, neurological diseases or be genetic. This is known as autonomic dysfunction.

- Constipation

- Unhealthy bacteria and/or yeasts in the small or large intestines; this is known as Small Intestinal Bacterial Overgrowth (SIBO) or Dysbiosis.

What can cause excess flatulence?

- Constipation

- Unhealthy bacteria in the large intestines (dysbiosis)

- A sudden change of diet, especially increasing the fiber content in the diet too quickly

- Eating sulfur containing foods (garlic, cabbage, eggs etc.)

What can be used to reduce excess intestinal gas?

Trial and error may be required, as some individuals are more sensitive to, or more troubled by gas, than others. Also the amount of gas or bloating a person has normally varies a lot and the experience can be quite subjective.

Treatment options for excess gas include:

- Reduce constipation –see page 40

- Drink more water in between meals

- Try reducing the amount of grain based fiber in your diet (bran, cereals, wholemeal breads etc) for 8 weeks and see what happens– for some people this can help a lot. For high fiber vegetables and fruits, use a high powered processor such as a Vitamix or Thermomix to blend your food to make it easier to digest.

- Eat smaller and more frequent meals

- Take digestive enzymes with meals

- If you have lost your gallbladder try taking ox bile capsules with meals

- Exclude gluten and dairy products and observe the effect – if no better after 4 months consult a dietitian to be checked for intolerance to foods high in FODMAPs – see page 133

- Try a grain free and legume free diet for 4 months (that means no wheat, rye, barley, oats, spelt, rice or corn and no beans, peas or lentils)

- Drink weaker coffee and tea

- Improve the amount of good bacteria in your gut by improving your diet, taking a probiotic and eating more fermented foods– see page 254

- Some doctors prescribe a nonabsorbable antibiotic such as rifaximin to reduce the growth of unhealthy bacteria in the small intestine – this can be useful in those who do not want to improve their diet

- Try natural antibiotics to reduce unhealthy bacteria in the gut – see pages 24 and 25.

- The herbal product for Irritable Bowel Syndrome (IBS) called Iberogast can be helpful and is quite popular in Europe and has been used for 50 years. It contains the combination of herbs Iberis amara, Angelica, Matricaria recuitita, Carum carvi, Silybum marianum, Melissa officianalis, Mentha piperitae, Chelidonium majus and Glycyrrhiza glabra

In severe cases the antispasmodic drugs such as mebeverine hydrochloride or hyoscine can help to reduce symptoms of excessive gas, especially if it is associated with abdominal cramps.

The old fashioned medication called Amitriptyline is often effective for IBS and abdominal cramps and diarrhea in those who suffer excess anxiety and/or insomnia. Only very small doses are required from 5 to 10mg at night.

Constipation

The normal frequency of bowel actions varies greatly between people. Ideally you should have from one to three bowel actions daily. They should be a brownish color, be soft and grainy and passed without undue straining. Many of my patients have told me that their stools have changed significantly after commencing the Liver Cleansing Diet and FiberTone powder. In particular they find that they are softer, easier to pass and longer in size. They may contain obvious pieces of undigested vegetables such as small parts of plant skins and small parts of leaves. This is a good sign because this increased fiber acts like a broom to cleanse the bowel walls.

Signs to worry about are red blood or a black color in the stools, or an obvious change in bowel habits from your normal pattern. It is good to look at each bowel action after you pass it to check for general appearance and color.

Effects of Chronic Constipation

If constipation becomes chronic and the bowel is not emptied effectively, waste products and feces will accumulate in loops, pockets, nooks and crannies in the bowel. In such places unfriendly bacteria and parasites may grow and this can cause a build up of toxins, which can affect general health. Toxins from the bowel may recirculate back to the liver. An overworked liver causes fatigue and poor general health.

The bowel may become inflated causing abdominal bloating, cramps and unpleasant gas and this is embarrassing for many people. If you have these problems it is wise to have a colonoscopy by a specialist doctor to exclude serious disease such as bowel cancer.

Chronic constipation can lead to hemorrhoids and anal fissures, which are painful and can bleed producing bright red blood. Constipation can lead to pockets in the bowel which may become inflamed – this is known as diverticulitis. Repetitive straining to pass hard feces can lead to a prolapsed rectum and/or fecal incontinence.

Laxatives

Laxatives are used to induce a bowel action and/or to prevent constipation.

Strong Laxatives

Some laxatives are very strong and may overstimulate the muscles of the bowel leading to irritation, colonic spasm and in the long-term, enlargement and permanent damage of the colon. For this reason they should not be used on a regular basis. Strong laxatives (cathartics) can be used occasionally for severe constipation. They include senna and cascara. Conventional laxatives are things like phenolphthalein and dioctyl sodium sulfosuccinate, and although they work swiftly, they can cause diarrhea and cramping. Strong laxatives can be habit forming.

Osmotic Laxatives

Osmotic laxatives such as magnesium sulphate (Epsom's salts), magnesium oxide and lactulose are a much safer alternative to cathartics, and I prefer to use them in cases of chronic constipation. Osmotic laxatives draw water into the colon and make the bowel actions soft and more liquid. They do not generally irritate the bowels. OsmoLax and Movicol are popular brands of osmotic laxatives that contain macrogol 3350 (polyethylene glycol).

Macrogol works by restoring the natural rhythm by using the body's own water to gently increase the frequency of bowel movements and to soften the stool. It relieves constipation because it causes the water it is taken with, to be retained in the bowel instead of being absorbed into the body. This increases the water content in the bowel, making the feces softer and easier to pass. Macrogol usually produces a bowel movement within 1 to 3 days. Macrogol can be used for children over 4 years of age as well as adults.

A slightly stronger effect from an osmotic laxative is obtained from combining magnesium oxide with senna leaf extract, peppermint leaf and cape aloe leaf. This product is known as Colon Cleanse and is available in capsule form. The usual dose is one to two capsules when constipated. See www.liverdoctor.com

Suppositories and Enemas

Suppositories and enemas are effective for sudden severe constipation of the lower bowel or fecal impaction. Some bowel therapists add herbs such as catnip or coffee to enemas to improve their cleansing effect. Fecal impaction means that hard feces get stuck in the rectum and lower colon, and obstruct the passage of softer feces higher up. This can lead to "spurious diarrhea" where the softer feces above the hard impacted feces liquefy and are then able to pass around the hard feces and it appears as though the patient has diarrhea when in reality they have severe constipation. This can occur in the very elderly, immobilized persons, over medicated patients or those with neurological diseases. This is why a doctor should perform a rectal examination in severely constipated patients. Fecal impaction may require manual extraction of the feces if an enema does not work. Thereafter regular enemas or colonic irrigations need to be given to prevent a recurrence.

Many people find that colonic irrigations are very beneficial in removing waste products from the bowel, and in experienced hands this is safe to do. If you have severe constipation, colonic irrigations from a registered practitioner every 2 to 4 weeks can be of great benefit.

However even if you have regular enemas or colonic irrigations you still need a high fiber diet and plenty of water, and if possible regular exercise. Enemas and/or colonic irrigations should not be performed in cases of inflammatory bowel disease, severe diverticulitis, or where there is a structural defect of the bowel. This is to avoid mechanical damage to the bowel in these cases.

Fiber

A high fiber diet is best obtained from eating plentiful vegetables and fruits. Grinding linseeds (flaxseeds), sunflower seeds and almonds into a fine powder can help stubborn constipation and can be eaten instead of bran. This powder mixture is known as LSA and can be purchased from supermarkets and health food stores or make it yourself in a grinder and store it in the freezer. Chia seeds are excellent for constipation and reduce bowel inflammation. Add chia seeds to smoothies or gluten free muesli.

Hemp seeds can be eaten regularly in salads and homemade muffins and smoothies and are excellent for constipation as they are high in fiber. You do not need to grind hemp seeds.

Fiber products can help constipation and the best known one is psyllium husks. An excellent gluten free fiber product called FiberTone is available from health food stores or on-line. FiberTone contains ginger powder, slippery elm bark, soy fiber, rice bran, peppermint powder, beetroot powder, broccoli powder, carob powder, spinach powder and tomato powder. FiberTone is a super food for the bowels; the dose is 1 or more teaspoons of FiberTone powder daily on cereal or in juice or water. FiberTone is suitable for all types of constipation as it acts like an "intestinal broom," sweeping the walls of the colon clean. Make sure that you drink plenty of pure water (2 liters daily) to help this powder do its work.

FiberTone can reduce irritable bowel syndrome and chronic constipation. It can also reduce bowel toxicity caused by fecal stagnation. FiberTone is also suitable for those who are allergic to gluten (found in wheat, oat, barley or rye). There are many types of fiber powders on the market that can increase the bulk of the feces and reduce constipation. These are safe to use in the long term and confer general health benefits. Other brands that I have found effective are, Normacol and Fybogel.

Diarrhea

Diarrhea is the opposite of constipation and refers to bowel actions that are too frequent and although this is an individual thing, if you have a bowel motion more than 4 times a day this is considered unusual. The average number of bowel actions in someone with a healthy bowel is one to two daily. In diarrhea the stool will be excessively watery and often explosive in nature with a sense of urgency to defecate. The stool may consist of only brownish to green water or may contain small amounts of feces mixed with mucus. There may be undigested food in the stools. There may be abdominal cramps and discomfort before and during the stool is passed.

Diarrhea disease is a leading cause of morbidity and mortality worldwide.

What are the causes of diarrhea?

• Inflammatory bowel diseases

• Irritable bowel syndrome

• Stress and anxiety may cause a "nervous bowel" which manifests as urgency to defecate and frequent need to defecate. The sufferer may not be able to lead a normal life, as things such as shopping, bus tours and holidays require an abundance of toilets. If toilets are not available considerable anxiety occurs and thus the patient becomes increasingly unable to participate in life. This problem of nervous diarrhea can be controlled with a small dose (5 to 10 mg) of the medication called Amitryptiline taken at night, several hours before sleep.

• Removal of the gallbladder may cause a reduction in bile flow during a meal which results in impaired absorption of dietary fats; this may cause fatty loose stools. This can be helped by taking a supplement of ox-bile capsules during the meal

• Diseases of the pancreas may cause impaired digestion and absorption of food resulting in diarrhea; this can be remedied with a supplement of pancreatic digestive enzymes during the meal

- Food intolerances such as lactose intolerance and FODMAP intolerance– see page 133

- Celiac disease or gluten intolerance – see page 83

- Bowel cancer can present as diarrhea, often alternating with constipation

- Infection of the bowel with parasites, viruses, fungi or bacteria. The most common cause of this is food contamination and this is known as food poisoning

Anyone with persistent and/or severe diarrhea should be referred to a gastroenterologist for a colonoscopy to find the specific cause. It is also important to do blood tests to detect inflammation, anemia or signs of infection.

It is vital to do tests on several fresh samples of the stools to try and find the type of micro-organism infecting the bowel. Most laboratories use conventional diagnostic tests – namely looking at the stool with a microscope and trying to grow (culture) various common disease causing micro-organisms on plates. The stool specimen is inoculated onto numerous media plates and incubated for 24 hours. The plates are then inspected for growth of colonies of micro-organisms. The laboratory technician must be skilled and experienced and a minimum of 48 to 72 hours is required before results can be reported. This delay in getting results may cause the doctor to panic and prescribe unnecessary antibiotics which are not correct for the specific infecting micro-organism. This type of testing with culture on plates has other limitations because some types of bacteria are difficult to grow and may not show up on the plates even though they are present in the stool. These failures to culture may occur in cholera, salmonella, shigella and campylobacter bacteria. Confusion can occur because normal (non-disease causing) bacteria in the intestinal flora can grow on the culture plate and resemble the colonies from disease causing bacteria. Parasites can be missed, as their protozoa are only intermittently shed in the stool and thus multiple stool samples are required. Final results such as sensitivity of the bacteria to antibiotics are obtained after 3 to 4 days so these tests are very time consuming and labor intensive. Thus microscopy and culture of the stool is not an exact science.

However all is not gloom and doom as exciting new technology for fast and accurate detection of micro-organisms causing bowel infections has just become available. This new technology is called Molecular Diagnostic Assays on stool specimens. It includes a technique known as multiplex PCR and enables rapid detection of multiple organisms including parasites, bacteria and viruses. The multiplex PCR testing is rapid and detects organisms that are impossible to culture and identify with plate techniques currently in use. The multiplex PCR technique is especially good for identifying viruses which may cause diarrhea. More pathology laboratories need to adopt this testing method for micro-organisms that cause bowel disease and diarrhea. If you suspect that you have a micro-organism causing your diarrhea, and this has remain undetected by conventional microscopy and plate culture tests, talk to your doctor about using this new PCR technique.

Megacolon

Megacolon is the term used for an abnormally enlarged colon. It is often associated with extra (redundant) loops of bowel. Megacolon can be congenital and is often hereditary, or can gradually develop over many years of poor diet, constipation and/or laxative abuse. If there is a very large amount of extra bowel, there may be huge redundant loops of bowel that trap food, which stagnates and putrefies inside them.

Megacolon is a mechanical problem and causes abdominal bloating, constipation, flatulence and pain.

The constipation produced is severe and it may be over a week before a bowel action eventuates. Understandably this is not completely solved with strong laxatives alone, and colonic irrigations are far more effective for megacolon.

Megacolon

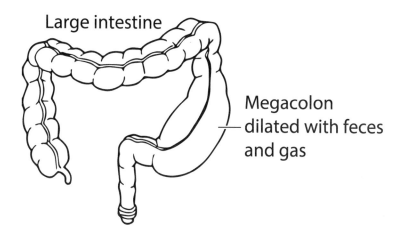

Large intestine

Megacolon dilated with feces and gas

In some people with severe constipation caused by a megacolon, there is damage to the nerves that supply the muscles in the colon and thus the contractions of the muscles are weak and do not move the feces along the colon. This type of nerve damage is commonly caused by diabetes, diseases of the brain and spinal cord, some medications and chemotherapy for cancer. In diabetics weight loss and blood sugar control can reduce nerve damage and thus constipation.

In people with severe constipation caused by megacolon and/or nerve damage, the use of regular enemas and/or colonic irrigations is essential.

A special X ray called a Barium Enema is able to diagnose Megacolon and shows the extra loops of unwanted bowel. In extreme cases the extra loops of bowel become huge, and great relief is achieved by surgically removing them and rejoining the healthy edges of the colon. The symptoms are relieved and the constipation cured. This surgical procedure is called a bowel resection and is best done by a surgeon who specializes in large bowel (colon) surgery. You can ask your general practitioner for a referral to such a specialist surgeon.

Case Histories and Testimonials

Dear Health Advisory Service,

I have been using a fiber powder for 10 weeks and I have noticed dramatic changes in my body. I had been a sufferer of abdominal bloating for 20 years and was most distressed to see my waistline getting larger every year. The bloating was much worse after eating and before my periods were due. I was unable to look nice in belts and my jeans would not fit, which made me very depressed. No matter what I tried to wear I looked awful and like a "middle aged frump." I have always been constipated with small hard stools that would not come out easily. I saw a specialist who performed a colonoscopy test on me and said that my bowel looked normal and was not enlarged. He diagnosed a lazy bowel!

I began using a powder called FiberTone and since using 3 teaspoons everyday and doubling my intake of water, my bowel actions have changed completely so that I now go three times every day and usually at the same time. The bowel actions are larger and much longer. My stomach has gradually gone down and I am now able to wear my jeans comfortably. I am so happy to think that I have found a natural solution, although I wished I had understood my problem years ago to avoid all the suffering.

Jacky Masters
Adelaide SA

Dear Dr. Cabot

I am a farmer who works with cattle and sheep and eat quite a lot of meat. I have been constipated for over 10 years and also suffered with irritable moods, hemorrhoids and itching around the anus. My wife finally got sick of my complaints and read your liver book. She then put me on two powders – one was a fiber powder and the other one was a potent magnesium powder. For the first 8 days it did not change much, but on the 9th day I had a huge bowel action that was well over one foot long and very offensive in smell. When I examined it I saw hundreds of small worms wriggling around in it and two long ones as well. I was disgusted and told my doctor who tested my bowel actions and found several varieties of parasites. I have been prescribed an anti-worm drug. I also used some natural Parasite Cleanse capsules and started eating garlic.

I have continued with the two powders for 9 months with very good results and now have 2 largish bowel actions daily without straining. The itch and bad moods have gone and I have lost 13 kilograms in weight. My wife wanted me to write to you and thank you for your excellent book

Joe McCormick
Perth WA

Inflammatory Bowel Disease

Inflammatory bowel disease (IBD) refers mainly to two chronic diseases that cause inflammation of the intestines: Ulcerative Colitis (UC) and Crohn's Disease (CD). Although UC and CD are different diseases, they often cause similar symptoms and share similar causes.

The severity of these diseases varies widely between individuals, with some having only mild symptoms whereas others have severe and disabling symptoms. Many researchers believe that inflammatory bowel disease is the result of an inherited predisposition that is triggered by an environmental agent (such as infection, food intolerance, antibiotic drugs and stress).There does not appear to be a direct predictable pattern of inheritance, but around 20% of patients with inflammatory bowel disease (IBD) have immediate family members with IBD.

Ulcerative Colitis (UC)

Ulcerative colitis (UC) is a disease of the large intestine (colon) and causes inflammation and ulceration of the inner lining (mucosa) of the colon and sometimes the rectum. In UC the bowel lining becomes ulcerated releasing blood, mucus and pus.

Inflammation of the rectum is called proctitis. Inflammation of the sigmoid colon (situated just above the rectum) is called sigmoiditis. Inflammation of the entire colon is called pan-colitis.

UC is autoimmune in origin; however it can flare up after emotional stress, antibiotic drugs and bacterial infections.

Inflammation of the bowel lining causes the colon to empty too frequently, resulting in diarrhea (sometimes explosive), cramping and flatulence. Bleeding from the bowel can occur and there may be up to 10 to 20 bowel actions daily which contain blood and mucus.. Weight loss, anemia, weakness, fever and dehydration often occurs during acute attacks.

Abscesses may form in the wall of the colon, which release infected pus into the colon. The colon may become very dilated and inflamed, which is a medical emergency known as toxic megacolon. Toxic megacolon occurs when inflammation spreads from the mucous lining through the remaining layers of the colon. The colon becomes paralyzed which causes it to swell so much that it can eventually burst. This is known as a bowel perforation, which requires emergency surgery. The overuse of certain drugs, particularly opiate painkillers and antispasmodics may increase the risk of toxic megacolon. This is why these drugs should be used with great care in UC.

UC begins most frequently in the 20 to 30 age group although older people and children occasionally develop this disease. A specialist gastroenterologist will carry out investigations such as direct visualization of the bowel lining using a fiber optic telescope (colonoscopy).

Treatment of Ulcerative Colitis

The diet will have to be adjusted according to the severity of symptoms. It needs to be high in easily absorbed forms of protein and carbohydrates. Protein powders made from pea protein, rice protein, whey, and egg white can be very helpful when solid foods cannot be tolerated.

High fiber foods may not be tolerated and indeed may often aggravate the diarrhea. In this situation, raw vegetable and fruit juices made freshly with a juice - extracting machine and diluted with water, can provide essential healing antioxidants. Some people will not need to dilute the raw juices while others have such an inflamed gut that they need to dilute the juice to have 2 parts pure water to one part juice. Drink 200 mls (7oz) of the raw juice every one to two hours. Glutamine powder can be mixed into these raw juices to provide more rapid healing of the ulcerated bowel lining.

During acute flare-ups of the UC, avoid high fiber cereals, seeds and nuts. Puree your fruits and vegetables after cooking them. Eat only small frequent meals.

Food preparation takes longer for those with inflammatory bowel disease because it is much better to eat your fruits and vegetables finely chopped or grated after they have been washed thoroughly. It is even better if you can afford to purchase a high powered food processor such as a Vitamix or Thermomix to blend whole fruits and vegetables into a whole-foods soup. These machines can make green smoothies with things such as avocado, kale, carrot, green apples, pears, ginger, mint, and cucumber.

You can add aloe vera to these smoothies or raw juices, but remove the spines first. See appendix page 262. Aloe vera can protect the lining of the bowel.

You can also add glutamine powder and/or slippery elm powder to the smoothies for an extra healing and soothing effect.

Green Smoothie Recipe

1 avocado (remove skin)

2 kale leaves

2 cabbage leaves

1 carrot

1 lime or lemon (remove skin)

2 apples

½ cucumber

6 mint leaves

2 tsp pure glutamine powder

2 aloe vera leaves (spines removed)

2 tsp slippery elm powder

Place in Vitamix and blend

All seeds and nuts should be finely ground in a coffee grinder or food processor. You do not have to grind hemp seeds, as these are soft and easily chewed and digested. You do not have to grind chia seeds as they soften when added to a fluid such as water or coconut milk. Chia seeds and hemp seeds are the most easily digested and non-irritating seeds for patients with inflammatory bowel disease and also contain anti-inflammatory omega 3 fatty acids.

It is important to avoid foods that may trigger attacks and everyone is different here. However I advise you to completely avoid gluten containing foods such as wheat, rye, barley and oats. Gluten has a high chance of aggravating autoimmune diseases such as UC and CD and this applies even if you are NOT diagnosed with celiac disease.

Some people will be much better off if they also avoid dairy products, such as cow's milk, butter, cream, ice cream and cheese. Margarine should also be avoided. Inflammatory bowel diseases often require both a gluten and dairy free diet long term in order to prevent recurrences.

Deep fried foods, very spicy foods, preserved, smoked and processed foods are better avoided. If enjoyed, red meat can be eaten but should be very fresh, very well cooked and eaten in small amounts.

Supplements of the fat-soluble vitamins (namely vitamins A, D, E, and K) should be taken regularly. Cod liver oil and grass fed lamb or calf liver (eaten as lamb's fry as a popular and healthy dish) are good sources of these vitamins. Grass fed liver can help to build up iron, protein and vitamin levels and is very healthy to eat if you have inflammatory bowel diseases. To see the benefits of eating liver see page 257 in appendix

If blood loss from the bowels has caused anemia, tablets of organic iron, vitamin C and folic acid should be given. Great benefit can be obtained from vitamin B 12 injections. Iron injections or transfusions may quickly overcome anemia and severe fatigue.

To reduce inflammation and speed up healing it is vital to provide nutritional supplements to balance the immune system. I recommend selenium 150 to 300mcg daily, Vitamin E 500IU twice daily, Vitamin C 500mg 2 to 3 times daily and vitamin D 3. The dose of vitamin D required will vary from 3000 to 5000 IU daily depending on what the blood level of vitamin D is. It is important to keep your blood level of vitamin D towards the high end of the normal range, because vitamin D is very beneficial for bowel and immune health. Take all these supplements at the beginning of meals. These nutritional supplements act as antioxidants and will reduce the risk of bowel cancer developing if they are taken long term. Selenium in particular is most beneficial for bowel cancer prevention and I recommend you visit www.seleniumresearch.com for more information.

I recommend you take Glutamine powder in a dose of 5 grams twice daily on a regular basis, as it has specific healing effects on the lining of the bowels – see page 31

Drug treatment is effective for the relief of acute symptoms in 70 - 80% of patients, and consists of anti-inflammatories, (such as sulfasalazine and steroids), antibiotics and antispasmodics. If the patient is using nutritional therapies in between attacks, the doses of steroid drugs can often be minimized and confined to much shorter time periods. The minerals magnesium and potassium will need to be replaced because diarrhea depletes these minerals.

Surgery becomes necessary in severe cases where intestinal perforation or obstruction has occurred.

Long term regular follow up is essential, because for patients who have had UC for over 10 years, the risk of colon cancer is increased. Patients who have both UC and the liver disease Sclerosing Cholangitis, may be at an even higher risk of colon cancer. These people should be screened with extra vigilance and must avoid gluten in the diet and take selenium supplements.

Some patients have told me that eating green bananas has been helpful in reducing UC and CD symptoms so this is worth bearing in mind, but I am not sure of the mechanism of action.

Probiotic supplements, such as lactobacillus-acidophilus etc, (see page 26) should be used regularly in those with inflammatory bowel disease (IBD). Fermented foods can also be used to promote healthy bacteria in the bowel and should be tried – see page 254

Crohn's Disease (CD)

Crohn's Disease (CD) is a severe inflammatory disease of the intestines, and like ulcerative colitis, it is autoimmune in origin. CD can affect any portion of the gastrointestinal tract from the esophagus to the anus. It most commonly attacks the last part of the small intestine (known as the ileum) where it joins the colon; this is known as the ileo-cecal area. See page 14. Crohn's Disease is sometimes called ileitis, which means inflammation of the ileum. In CD the inflammation of the bowel can be so deep that all layers of the bowel are affected. Eventually scarring may cause narrowing and/or blockage of the intestinal tube (lumen).

Symptoms of CD can include abdominal pain, fever, anemia, blood in the feces, watery and/or bloody bowel actions, chronic diarrhea, weight loss and fissures in the anal area.

CT scans and MRI scans reveal a thickened, scarred and narrowed intestinal wall. The feces (stools) will often test positive for blood and pus. The feces should also be cultured to detect unhealthy bacteria.

A colonoscopy will need to be done to assess severity of the disease – see page 265

Treatment of Crohn's Disease (CD)

The diet must be adjusted according to the severity of the symptoms and is similar to the diet discussed for ulcerative colitis. The absorption of nutrients from the inflamed small bowel lining may be poor and it is usual to require a diet high in easily absorbed forms of protein and carbohydrates. Small frequent meals are better tolerated. Gluten containing foods and dairy products should be avoided completely, as these foods will greatly aggravate CD.

When the bowel is inflamed, high fiber foods are not tolerated well, and many foods such as fruits and vegetables must be pureed in a blender. A Vitamix or Thermomix are wonderful utensils, as they can make whole food smoothies and soups. See page 51 for a green smoothie recipe.

British researchers have discovered that two-thirds of patients with CD, harbor bacteria in their intestine which are strikingly similar to the bacteria that causes Johne's disease in cattle. They also found this bacteria in pasteurized cow's milk and they have found it to be very resilient to destruction, surviving in manure, soil and waterways. This is another good reason to avoid dairy products if you have CD and the best milks to consume are almond, rice or coconut milk.

Supplements of potassium and magnesium are needed after attacks of diarrhea.

If the ileum is diseased, be aware that vitamin B 12 deficiency may occur, and it is important to have a blood test to check your vitamin B 12 level. If B 12 levels are low, injections of vitamin B 12 should be given every 4 to 6 weeks.

Deficiencies of fat-soluble vitamins may also occur, which will reduce the ability of the bowel to heal. For this reason it is wise to take supplements of the fat-soluble vitamins, namely vitamins A, D, E and K. These can be taken individually and are also present in cod liver oil, lamb and calf liver and dark green and orange colored vegetables. To see the benefits of eating liver see page 257 in appendix.

Spinach, kale and cabbage are excellent to provide antioxidants to heal an inflamed intestine. If you do not like the taste of cod liver oil, this is easily overcome by using capsules of cod liver oil, which can be taken just before meals. Take 2 capsules just before every meal.

It is not uncommon to find that people with CD have problems digesting and absorbing nutrients from food. Taking digestive enzymes with every meal can help this – see page 22

Drugs are required for acute attacks and consist of antibiotics and anti-inflammatories (such as Sulfasalazine, and Azulfadine and steroids) and anti-spasmodics.

During a severe attack of CD or UC, hospitalization with intravenous hydration, intravenous steroids, total parenteral nutrition (nutrients given intravenously), and transfusions of packed red blood cells is often life saving. If these severe inflammatory bowel diseases are not controlled properly, complications such as intestinal obstruction, severe hemorrhaging, abscesses, infection, fistulas, perforation of the bowel or toxic swelling of the entire colon (toxic megacolon) may supervene.

There is a slightly higher risk of cancer of the small intestine and anus in suffers of CD. In those with longstanding (over 8 years) inflammatory disease of the colon, whether it be due to UC or CD, it is generally agreed by the experts that a regular screening colonoscopy should be done. This is to look for early signs of cancer. If multiple precancerous lesions are found most experts recommend removal of the colon (colectomy).

To reduce the risk of cancerous lesions developing in the bowel it is important to follow a gluten free diet. I also advise a dairy free or low dairy diet.

It is also essential to supplement with the antioxidants selenium, vitamin C, vitamin E and vitamin D. These antioxidants have been proven to exert a protective effect against many types of cancers, including bowel cancer. See www.liverdoctor.com/free-ebooks/

Another excellent source of these antioxidants is raw vegetable juices such as carrot, beetroot, celery, apple, citrus, ginger, spinach, kale, cabbage, and any green leafy herbs. Add one teaspoon of glutamine powder to your juices and smoothies and drink twice daily, but if you are too busy, even once a day will make a big difference. Glutamine is an excellent supplement for people with Crohn's disease, as it not only provides a fuel for the intestinal cells it also repairs intestinal inflammation.

Raw juices can be made freshly every day with a juice extractor or you can make a week's supply and freeze the juice immediately after making it. Freeze in glass jars left over from the supermarket and leave 1cm (1/2 inch) at the top for expansion during freezing. These juices contain powerful anti-cancer phyto-nutrients.

Some patients have told me that eating green bananas has been helpful in reducing UC and CD symptoms so this is worth bearing in mind, but I am not sure of the mechanism of action.

Probiotic supplements such as lactobacillus-acidophilus etc, (see page 26) should be used regularly in those with inflammatory bowel disease (IBD). Fermented foods can also be used to promote healthy bacteria in the bowel and should be tried – see page 254

Problems with the anus

The anus is the end of the digestive tract and complaints in this area are common.

An itchy anus is very unpleasant and can cause considerable distress from repeated scratching, especially when the area becomes warmer in bed at night. Sweating and tight underpants can also aggravate anal itching. An itchy anus is often caused by dermatitis or eczema in this area and the standard treatment is a cortisone cream to suppress the inflammation. This treatment is very effective but does not treat the cause, as it is only suppressing the inflammation. If the anus and its surrounding skin is inflamed it is often associated with inflammation in the rectum and colon.

To correct this inflammation it is necessary to improve the diet and it is important to reduce sugar and gluten in the diet and indeed a trial of a gluten free and sugar free diet is most worthwhile. Increase the amount of fresh vegetables and raw fruits in the diet. Improve the population of healthy bacteria in the colon by taking a probiotic supplement and consuming more fermented foods in your diet – see page 254

The anus may become dry and inflamed because of a lack of healthy fats in the diet so increase your consumption of oily fish, coconut oil, ground flaxseeds, hemp seeds and organic free range eggs. Cracks known as fissures can form in the anus and these can be painful and bleed. Fissures can be improved by overcoming constipation by drinking more water and increasing fiber and omega 3 fatty acids in the diet. To heal fissures supplements of zinc, selenium, vitamin E and vitamin C are needed.

An inexpensive cream called "Castor Oil and Zinc Cream" can be applied to the area afflicted by fissures and/or dermatitis and this is soothing and promotes healing. If the pain from the fissures is very acute and makes it hard to pass a bowel action, a local anesthetic cream can be applied to the fissures.

Intestinal parasites (such as worms or candida) can lead to anal itching and a stool specimen should be obtained and cultured to check for these parasites. To overcome intestinal parasites see pages 24 and 25.

If the itching and irritation of the anus and its surrounding skin has been present for many years a condition known as lichen sclerosis may be found on examination of the area. This can be confirmed with a biopsy of the affected area. In women the lichen sclerosis may affect the vulva and perineum as well as the anus, and these patients complain of discomfort, dryness and itching in all these areas. Lichen sclerosis is an autoimmune disorder and the chronic inflammation can lead to thinning, scarring and distortion of these parts of the skin and mucous membranes, and can eventually become malignant (develop cancerous changes). In patients with lichen sclerosis I recommend a gluten free diet and an increased intake of healthy fats in the diet. Raw juicing with green leafy vegetables and citrus fruits, and supplements of zinc, selenium and vitamin C and E are essential. Hormonal creams containing oestriol and testosterone can help to heal lichen sclerosis in menopausal women. Steroid creams can reduce the severe inflammation and provide relief from pain and itching in the vulva, perineum and anus.

Irritable Bowel Syndrome

This common problem has been known in the past by several different names such as "spastic colon" or "nervous bowel". Irritable Bowel Syndrome (IBS) means an irritability of the bowel and this can affect any area of the digestive tract. A syndrome is a group of symptoms and signs that occur together and produce a typical pattern of a specific disorder.

Classic symptoms of IBS are:

- Abdominal pain- this may vary from dull aching, swollen pressure, cramping, or sharp in nature. The pains are usually intermittent and may disappear for long periods of time.

- Irregular pattern of the bowel actions – constipation or diarrhea, or constipation alternating with diarrhea.

- Other symptoms may include belching, bloating, reduced appetite and excessive gas (flatulence).

The exact cause of IBS is unknown and is likely to be due to several factors operating together. To understand these factors, see causes of Bowel Dysfunction on page 15

In all sufferers the end result is a disordered rhythm in the muscles of the gastrointestinal tract. Normal intestinal contractions are called peristalsis, and consist of "segmental contractions" and "propulsive contractions". Segmental contractions churn and mix intestinal contents while propulsive contractions move the intestinal contents forwards on their way to the rectum for expulsion. Exaggerated segmental contractions may cause cramps, bloating and constipation. If the forward movement of intestinal contents decreases, the bowel actions may become harder and more compressed. This makes them harder to pass.

If the propulsive contractions are exaggerated, explosive watery diarrhea may occur. This may cause an urgent desire to defecate, which can be very stressful, if a toilet is unavailable.

Spastic colon

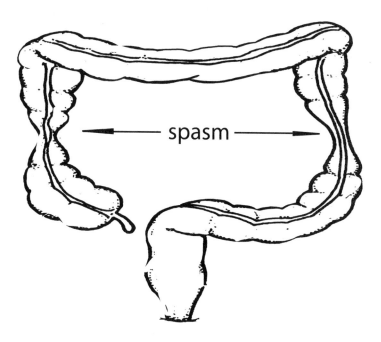

Treatment of Irritable Bowel Syndrome

- Set aside enough time to eat, and eat in a relaxed atmosphere. Think pleasant positive thoughts while eating and chew your food thoroughly. If you take sufficient time to eat, the digestive enzymes from the salivary glands in your mouth will be able to mix well with the food.

- Do not eat with people who make you feel emotionally disturbed. It may be who you are eating with, rather than what you are eating, that is causing your IBS.

- Do not talk excessively while eating as you may swallow excessive gas with the food, which will cause bloating.

- Avoid drinking large amounts of liquid with the meal, as this will dilute digestive enzymes.

- If you have a weak digestive system take digestive enzymes in the middle of your meal and sip one to two tablespoons of organic apple cider vinegar diluted in 3 tablespoons of water during the meal.

- Avoid carbonated (fizzy) beverages or chewing gum or mints after eating, as this will increase the gas in your stomach.

- Do not eat your food too rapidly because this will tend to cause overeating. This is because the hormone cholecystokinin is released into the bloodstream from the small intestine in response to a meal. It then travels to the appetite control center in the brain and tells you when you have eaten enough. If you rush down (gulp) your food there is insufficient time for the cholecystokinin hormone to switch off your hunger and you will probably overeat. It is far better to be a gourmet than a gourmand, and really experience the delicate flavors in every mouthful of your food.

- Avoid excessive intake of alcohol.

- Consult a nutritionist to detect food intolerances to specific foods – the most common foods to cause IBS are gluten, dairy products and foods high in FODMAPs – see page 133. Eliminate gluten containing foods for 3 months to see if this cures your IBS.

- Take a good probiotic supplement to increase amounts of healthy bacteria in the bowel – see page 26. Include more fermented foods in the diet – see page 254

One of my patients had been a very obese woman or as she said a "yo-yo dieter." She told me that she had lost more than six hundred pounds in weight over the last 20 years and put more than that back on! She finally understood the importance of the liver in fat metabolism after reading my books, which allowed her to understand that "oils ain't oils." She started to replace damaged fats like margarine and deep fried foods with healthy sources of fats such as fish, lean veal, eggs, lamb, hemp seeds, avocados, tahini paste, coconut oil and cold pressed olive oil. She changed her habits from eating heaps of sugary foods to different types of flavors using natural condiments such as fresh garlic, coriander, curry powder, tomato paste, ginger and pesto sauces. She was able to feel satisfied after these foods because she was not on a low fat diet. Rather she was on the right fat diet, which is why she is now successful in keeping her weight and IBS under control.

Foods that may worsen IBS:

- Preserved and processed foods containing high amounts of sugar, artificial colorings, preservatives or flavorings.

- Gluten containing foods (wheat, rye, barley and oats) can cause IBS.

- The sugar found in milk, which is called lactose, may cause IBS. Lactose intolerance results from a deficiency of the intestinal enzyme called lactase. Lactase is required to break down lactose into the simple sugars called glucose and galactose. Lactose intolerance is more common in Asian people and also becomes more frequent with age and after intestinal infections. If you are lactose intolerant, but cannot live without dairy products, it is possible to obtain cow's milk that is processed to be lactose free. It is also possible to obtain tablets or drops containing the enzyme lactase, which digests lactose, and this can be taken with meals containing dairy products.

- Some types of sweeteners and flavorings can cause IBS, such as sugar alcohols (sorbitol, xylitol, maltitol and erythritol) or aspartame or monosodium glutamate (MSG).

- Fructose is the sugar found in all fruits and is used as a sweetener in some soft drinks. If you are intolerant to fructose (fruit sugar) you may find that juices of fruits and/or vegetables cause symptoms of IBS. This is because the juices concentrate the fructose. In this case you can dilute the juices with water, (2 parts water to 1 part juice is a good starting point) or rely on eating the whole fruits and vegetables. The extra fiber from the whole vegetable or fruit is more beneficial than pure juices in sufferers of IBS.

- Certain vegetables (such as cruciferous vegetables, garlic or onions) may give you unpleasant gas and bloating. This can be avoided by lightly cooking them and then blending them in a food processor or turning them into an Italian vegetable soup (minestrone).

If you suspect food intolerances to be causing your IBS, keep a food diary, see page 157, which lists the foods you ate that day and the digestive symptoms experienced afterwards. Do this for 8 weeks and then go back over it and you may find some telltale patterns.

Check the Fiber Content of your Diet

Your diet should be providing 30 to 40 grams of fiber every day. If your diet is currently low in fiber you should increase your daily fiber intake gradually to allow your intestines to adjust. Otherwise you may suffer with bloating and excessive gas.

By gradually increasing dietary fiber you will overcome many of the symptoms of irritable bowel syndrome. A high fiber intake has also been proven to reduce your chances of bowel cancer.

To help you increase fiber intake here is a list of high-fiber foods

Fiber Content of Foods

Vegetables	Dietary Fiber (grams)
Asparagus, 1 cup	3.1
Beans, 1 cup pinto	5.3
Beans, 1 cup green	2.1
Beans, 1 cup kidney	5.8
Beetroot, 1 cup	2.5
Broccoli, 1 cup	3.0
Brussels sprouts, 1 cup	2.8
Cabbage, 1 cup	2.8
Cauliflower, 1 cup	1.8
Lettuce, 1 cup	0.5
Onion, 1 cup	2.1
Carrots, 1 cup	3.0
Peas, 1 cup	5.0
Potato, 1 medium baked	3.0
Spinach, 1 cup cooked	5.7
Tomatoes, 1 medium	1.4
Turnips, 2/3 cup	2.0
Sweet corn,1/2 cup	4.7
Zucchini, 1 cup	2.7

Fruits	Dietary Fiber (grams)
Apple, 1 medium	2.8
Banana, 1 medium	1.8
Berries, 1 cup	2.0
Cherries, 16 large	1.0
Figs, 2 dried	6.4
Grapes, 15	2.0
Orange, 1 medium	3.2
Peach, 1 medium	2.2
Pineapple, 1/3 cup	0.5
Plums, 2 small	1.5
Prunes, 6 medium	2.0
Strawberries, 12 medium	2.0

Grains/Cereals/Nuts	Dietary Fiber (grams)
Corn flakes, 1 cup	2.0
Wheat bran, 1 cup	2.5
Shredded wheat, 1 wafer	2.7
Rice, (brown) cooked, 1/2 cup	2.4
Rice, (white) cooked, 1 cup	0.1
Brazil nuts, 1/3 cup	2.9
Peanuts, 1 cup	6.6
Sunflower seeds, 1 cup	8.0

Bread	Dietary Fiber (grams)
Wholegrain, (wheat) 1 slice	1.4
White bread, 1 slice	0.5
Rye bread, 1 slice	1.0

Dietary fiber is found in two different forms:

1. Soluble fiber which dissolves in water such as mucilages, gums and pectins.

2. Insoluble fiber which does not dissolve in water such as cellulose, most hemicelluloses and lignans.

Vegetables, fruits, grains, legumes and seeds contain a mixture of these two types of fiber. In the colon fiber is acted upon by friendly bacteria, which causes fermentation of the fibrous food remnants in the colon. This helps to make the stools soft, moist and larger so they are easier to pass and also travel along the large bowel easily without requiring undue contractions from the bowel. Beans contain gums, which are a good source of water-soluble fibers. Sweet corn contains a mixture of fibers and is an excellent food for those wanting to improve their bowel patterns. Raw fruits and vegetables are an excellent cleansing source of both types of fiber.

I have had several patients who have complained of excessive gas and bloating after increasing their intake of beans, seeds and raw vegetables. Remember to increase these things very gradually, using only small amounts to begin with. You can also take one to two tablespoons of organic apple cider vinegar mixed in water and sip it slowly during the meal. Another tip that often works is to use digestive enzymes during the meal.

Many suffers of IBS do not drink enough water, which will increase symptoms of constipation and flatulence. I have found that increasing water intake to at least 2 liters daily will overcome many of the symptoms of IBS. Drink this water in between meals.

For very acute and severe attacks of IBS that can be precipitated by stress or really letting go of your diet, medication may be needed. This may require the use of drugs to stop spasm in the muscles of the bowel (antispasmodics), laxatives for severe constipation or drugs to stop diarrhea. You should see your doctor for these things and self-medication is not advisable. For people with explosive diarrhea that is hard to control a small dose (5 to 10mg) of a medication called Amitryptiline taken at night can prevent this.

Prolapsed Colon

The transverse colon goes from the right side to the left side of the abdominal cavity and is made of muscular tissue. If the transverse colon becomes overloaded with feces, the force of gravity will cause it to droop down or prolapse into the lower abdominal and pelvic cavities.

Prolapsed Colon

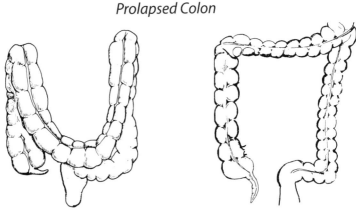

Prolapsed Colon   Healthy Colon

A prolapsed transverse colon will put pressure on the lower abdominal and pelvic organs. Weakness of the abdominal muscles, and excessive fat inside the abdominal cavity will further increase the downward forces upon the transverse colon. The chronically prolapsed transverse colon may become enlarged and twisted, producing extra loops of colon, which is known as redundant bowel. Redundant bowel is useless bowel and acts like a stagnant reservoir for fermentation of feces.

This leads to an increase in unfavorable bacteria in the bowel and absorption of toxins from the bowel into the blood stream; these toxins are carried back to the liver. This process is known as autointoxication and can cause severe flatulence and chronic ill health.

To reduce this problem it is vital to follow a regular exercise program including abdominal exercises, brisk walking and swimming. Regular Yoga and Pilates can be especially helpful for prolapsed colon. Massage of the abdominal area in the direction of the movement of the feces can be very helpful if done regularly. Avoidance of constipation is essential and regular colonic irrigations can help a lot.

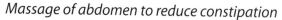

Massage of abdomen to reduce constipation

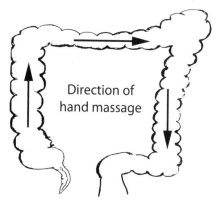

Direction of hand massage

Problems in the mouth

Bad breath, mouth ulcers and dry mouth

The mouth is known as the oral cavity and is the beginning of the digestive tract. Common problems in this area include bad breath, mouth ulcers and dry mouth with lack of saliva.

Bad Breath

Bad breath is known as halitosis and is a common and embarrassing problem.

The most common causes of bad breath include:

- Poor dental health with broken or infected teeth

- Gum disease known as periodontal disease

- Dry mouth and lack of saliva – this is known as xerostomia

- Mouth ulcers on the gums, cheeks and tongue

- A coated tongue

- Sinus infections with post nasal drip of infected secretions down the back of the throat

- Smoking cigarettes

- Unhealthy bacteria in the stomach such as infection with helicobacter pylori – see page 71

A two week detox, or a four day water fast, can improve the population of bacteria in your gut and I highly recommend this to improve your breath and the taste in your mouth– see page 251 Take a good probiotic supplement and eat more raw fruits and vegetables and avoid sugar.

A solution of 3% hydrogen peroxide can be obtained on a script from your doctor and 3 drops can be put in a small glass of water and swilled around the mouth and spat out. The hydrogen peroxide will kill the bacteria that lead to plaque and gum disease and reduce bad breath.

Gargling with colloidal silver also reduces bad bacteria in the mouth and I recommend you gargle with 2 tablespoons and spit it out after wards. Good dental hygiene is imperative and flossing, tooth picks or dental brushes should be used after eating.

Grow some fresh mint in your garden or pots and chew it regularly to improve your breath.

Dry Mouth

Dry mouth can be associated with dry eyes and may be a sign of an autoimmune disorder called Sjogren's Syndrome where damage occurs to the salivary glands and the mucous lining of the oral cavity. This can be helped by following a gluten free diet and taking supplements of omega 3 fatty acids found in oily fish, fish oil and krill oil supplements, chia seeds, hemp seeds and ground flaxseeds. Increase your intake of healthy fats from avocados, coconut oil and cold pressed olive oil. The mouth rinse Biotene can help to reduce dry mouth symptoms. Biotene is a dental hygiene product which is available in a number of forms, including toothpaste, mouthwash and cream. The toothpaste contains sodium monofluorophosphate and all Biotene products contain enzymes including glucose oxidase, lactoferrin, lactoperoxidase and lysozyme. Biotène can reduce the rate of recurrence of dental plaque but does not significantly reduce the count of Streptococcus mutans, which is the cause of the formation of dental plaque. This is where the hydrogen peroxide and colloidal silver can help to kill these bad bacteria. Biotene is available at your local pharmacy

Mouth Ulcers

Mouth ulcers are often recurrent and are very painful as there are many nerve endings in the mouth. They can be prevented by following a gluten free diet and taking supplements of zinc, selenium, vitamin C and vitamin D. It is also important to increase the amount of omega fatty acids in the diet as for dry mouth and dry eyes syndrome. Raw juicing with vegetables such as ginger, carrot, mint, parsley, lemon or lime and cabbage can prevent mouth ulcers by improving the immune system. You will need to keep these things up regularly and long term or the ulcers will recur.

The appearance of the tongue gives many clues as to the health of the digestive tract and liver. A thick white coating usually indicates an overgrowth of candida and perhaps other unhealthy yeasts and bacteria in the oral cavity and intestines. To overcome candida see page 120

A cracked and red tongue indicates inflammation and is a sign of a dysfunctional liver. It can also indicate deficiency of B vitamins and vitamin C.

Some people have a tongue with well defined patterns of different textures and color which resemble a map and this is known as a geographical tongue. If this is tender it indicates a dysfunctional liver. To improve your liver function you can take a liver formula containing milk thistle, selenium, taurine, vitamin C, B vitamins, folinic acid, zinc, green tea extract and N-Acetyl-Cysteine (NAC). LivaTone Plus contains all these ingredients in one capsule.

Peptic Ulcers

These types of ulcers refer to those found in the stomach (gastric ulcers), or first section of the small intestine (duodenal ulcers). These ulcers look like raw areas of erosion and can be small or large, singular or multiple, and deep or superficial, see diagram below.

I well remember when I worked in a missionary hospital in the Himalayan foothills during the early 1980s, that a very large number of young to middle aged Indian males came to the hospital with acute rupture of peptic ulcers. This is a life-threatening emergency and needless to say a good percentage of them perished from the peritonitis that ensued after rupture. I finally discovered that the cause was the home made alcoholic brew that was part of their culture in that area. This combined with a marginal diet and smoking Indian "bidi" cigarettes had made them vulnerable to ulceration of the stomach and duodenum

Peptic Ulcer

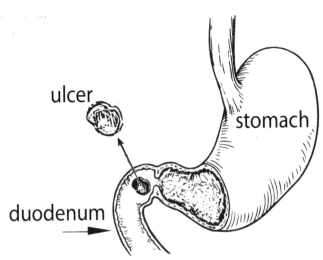

Symptoms of peptic ulcers can range from "hunger pains" to an intense burning pain in the center of the upper abdomen that will make you double up in agony. This pain is usually worse at night and when the stomach is empty. Stress can also bring on an attack. Eating food and drinking milk will often temporarily deaden the pain.

Factors that can cause or exacerbate peptic ulcers are stress, poor diet, missing meals, smoking, alcohol excess, analgesic drugs and anti-inflammatory drugs (both non-steroidal and steroidal varieties).

Helicobacter Pylori

In 1982 a breakthrough in the understanding of peptic ulcer disease resulted from the research of an Australian doctor, Dr Barry Marshall. He had discovered a causal link between stomach infection with the bacteria called Helicobacter Pylori, and the development of peptic ulceration. Initially his theories were viewed with great skepticism, however after numerous worldwide studies it is now proven categorically, that infection with this nasty little helicopter shaped bacteria is associated with inflammation of the stomach and duodenum, which can lead to ulceration.

Tests such as a breath test are available to detect infection with Helicobacter Pylori and your doctor can arrange these tests for you. If this infection is found, antibiotic treatment may be required and is usually quite successful. However like all chronic parasitic infections, helicobacter pylori tends to recur when your defenses are down or your diet is high in sugar and processed foods. You do not want to stay on antibiotics forever because they may create new problems for you such as candida, dysbiosis, allergies or liver problems. This is why nutritional medicine is so important in the treatment of chronic infections such as Helicobacter Pylori.

In those with peptic ulcers the diet should consist of small frequent meals that contain plenty of vegetables and fruits. During acute attacks it may be more comfortable to eat only homemade soups (vegetables and legumes), steamed vegetables and fish and rice.

"Smoothies" made with coconut milk, banana, berries, papaya, glutamine powder and slippery elm powder are soothing and healing and small amounts can be drunk regularly throughout the day. Bananas contain phospholipids that are surface active and needed to maintain the protective layer on the stomach mucosa. Raw vegetable juices containing cucumber, carrot, celery, mint and apple are beneficial for their healing and soothing properties. Raw cabbage juice has traditionally been used to heal ulcers. It is effective, despite its taste, because it contains substances which have powerful ulcer healing properties. Cabbage is also high in the liver amino acid glutamine, which stimulates mucin synthesis to enhance mucosal healing. The cabbage juice can be mixed with the other juices mentioned here to improve its flavor.

Natural Remedies for Peptic Ulcers

• Slippery Elm powder stirred into coconut, almond or rice milk can be used as desired, as it is free of side effects.

• Vitamins A and E, and the minerals zinc and selenium will speed healing and improve the health of the mucosal lining.

• Herbal teas such as chamomile, arrowroot, marshmallow, liquorice and golden seal are soothing and healing. These can be sweetened with a little stevia or Nature Sweet Sugar Substitute if desired.

• Aloe Vera plant juice/gel or liquid can be blended in your smoothies or juices and has specific healing effects on peptic ulcers – see page 262

• Smoothies are excellent for those with peptic ulcers – see recipe page 153

• The amino acid glutamine is excellent for those with peptic ulcers or gastritis. Glutamine serves as a source of fuel for cells lining the intestines, and without it these cells waste away. Glutamine helps to protect the lining of the gastrointestinal tract known as the mucosa and maintains the health of the mucosa. Digestion and normal metabolic function of the intestines are dependent upon adequate amounts of glutamine. Glutamine is most effective when taken as a powder of pure glutamine with a concentration of 5 grams per teaspoon. Use half to one teaspoon of this powder, two or three times daily.

• There are natural antibiotics which can be purchased, which include the following ingredients: phellodendron, oregano leaf oil, thyme leaf oil and clove oil. The recommended dosage is to take 2 capsules twice daily with food, but it may be necessary to take it 3 times daily. One such product is called BactoClear; they are enteric coated to ensure the capsule is delivered to the small intestine. These natural antibiotics help to keep down the population of Helicobacter Pylori and other unhealthy bacteria in the stomach and small intestine which can cause peptic ulcers.

Gastro-Esophageal Reflux Disease (GERD)

This is a common problem and is known by the acronym GERD and stands for Gastro-Esophageal Reflux Disease. Over time the reflux of stomach acid causes reflux esophagitis (meaning inflammation of the esophagus). GERD is also called "heartburn," although it has nothing to do with the heart. It may produce a burning discomfort behind the sternum which may extend up into the throat or may not produce any symptoms. If reflux occurs during sleep when you are horizontal, you may awake with a sore throat or a husky voice and an irritating cough.

GERD is caused by the acid contents of the stomach regurgitating or flowing backwards into the esophagus. The lining of the esophagus is not designed to handle these high acid conditions, which lead to inflammation, and in severe cases, scarring and ulceration of the lining of the esophagus.

The stomach produces a lot of hydrochloric acid during eating and for good reason, because without it, you cannot digest proteins efficiently and you will not absorb calcium and other minerals from foods.

There is a circular muscle around the lower esophagus, which divides it from the stomach, and this normally remains contracted to prevent back flow of stomach acid. During swallowing this muscle normally relaxes, allowing food to pass from the esophagus into the stomach, after which it should remain contracted. If this circular muscle becomes weakened or too relaxed, reflux can occur after meals.

If you are overweight and/or have a fatty liver, this will cause too much pressure on the stomach, and reflux becomes worse. If you eat a lot of sugar or refined carbohydrates such as cakes and biscuits, this will feed unhealthy bacteria in the stomach and this will make your stomach inflamed and overly sensitive to the hydrochloric acid. Thus is it vital to avoid sugary foods.

In some people with reflux there is also a hernia (protrusion) of the upper part of the stomach through the diaphragm into the lower chest. See diagram page 270 This is called a hiatus hernia and can be hereditary and is more common with age and in those who are overweight. A hiatus hernia will impair the function of the circular muscle around the lower esophagus. This increases reflux and heartburn symptoms. These symptoms are much worse after eating a large meal and while bending over.

If you suffer with long standing esophageal reflux it is important to see your gastroenterologist regularly, because prolonged exposure of the fragile esophageal mucosa to acid can result in an increased risk of esophageal cancer, severe scarring and narrowing (stricture formation). The passage inside the esophagus can become so narrowed that a stricture develops. This causes difficulty in swallowing normal amounts of food and results in pain, obstruction, or vomiting up the food that gets stuck. Surgery to enlarge the lower esophagus may then become necessary.

In severe cases of reflux esophagitis, medications to block stomach acid production should be taken if natural therapies fail. These are very effective and examples of these drugs are cimetidine, famotidine, nizatidine, rantidine and omeprazole.

Antacid drugs

The most common drugs used to reduce acid production by the stomach are Proton Pump Inhibitors (PPIs) and Histamine 2 Receptor Antagonists. Examples of these drugs are esomeprazole and pantoprazole.

These drugs are amongst the world's most commonly prescribed drugs. They are used to medically treat gastric and duodenal ulcers and Gastro-Esophageal Reflux Disease (GERD). They may also be used to prevent stomach and duodenal ulcers associated with the use of non-steroidal anti-inflammatory drugs. PPIs reduce the production of stomach acid by blocking the enzyme in the wall of the stomach that produces acid.

There may be side effects from using these drugs long term and they include –

• An increased risk of developing osteoporosis (bone loss). High dose therapy with PPIs and/or Histamine -2 Receptor Blocker drugs can significantly increase the risk of hip fractures.

• Impaired absorption of minerals

• Kidney damage

• An increased risk of vitamin B 12 deficiency – this can be serious as B 12 is required for the nervous system to function normally. In people taking antacid drugs, an annual test for vitamin B 12 blood levels should be done. If vitamin B 12 levels are found to be low, B12 injections must be given every 6 weeks.

Long term side effects of these drugs have even proven to be fatal in some extreme cases. An article in the JAMA Internal Medicine 2013 cites a 50% increased death risk post-discharge from hospital in elderly patients who have been given too many drugs (known as poly-pharmacy), including the proton pump inhibitor drugs. It is best to use the smallest dose of these drugs possible to try to avoid these potentially serious side effects.

Natural therapies and weight control can often bring great relief to those with excess stomach acidity or reflux.

Try these simple techniques to reduce reflux -.

• If you are overweight, it is vital to lose weight, and the best way to do this is with a diet low in sugar and grains, and high in vegetables and protein.

• Meal sizes should be small, as large meals increase pressure inside the stomach.

• Do not drink with your meals and confine your fluid intake to between meals.

• Do not eat food during the 3 hours before retiring to bed. It is wise to drink alkaline beverages during this time such as herbal teas, aloe vera juice or celery, mint, cucumber and carrot juice.

- Elevate the top of your bed by 6 to 8 inches by placing blocks under the head of the bed or purchase an electric bed with an adjustable slope angle.

- Avoid tight fitting clothes around the middle and do not bend over after meals.

- Avoid excessive coffee and alcohol and preserved foods. Some people find that spicy food such as chili or curry will aggravate symptoms, so trial and error is required.

- A diet low in sugar and deep fried foods will reduce symptoms of heartburn and reflux.

- Consume a diet high in vegetables to reduce the symptoms of heartburn.

- Raw juices or green smoothies can help to alkalinize the stomach between meals. Alkaline juices or smoothies contain plenty of green produce such as green apples, celery, cucumber, mint, parsley and fennel combined with carrot; these foods alkalinize your gut thereby reducing excess stomach acidity.

- If you are taking long term antacid drugs such as PPIs, it is wise to sip organic apple cider vinegar during your meals to increase acid for the digestive processes. Dilute 1 to 2 tablespoons of the apple cider vinegar in 3 tablespoons of water and sip slowly during your meals.

Natural Supplements to reduce reflux:

- Magnesium Powder (such as Magnesium Ultrapotent) in a dose of ½ teaspoon twice daily in water or vegetable juices to strengthen the muscular valve between the esophagus and stomach.

- Slippery elm powder and/or Aloe Vera juice mixed in vegetable juice or coconut, rice or almond milk, can reduce acidity; take it in between meals. To make your own aloe vera juice see page 262

- Selenium is an essential daily supplement for those with chronic reflux because it is a powerful antioxidant that helps to prevent cancerous changes in the esophagus.

• Soothing herbal teas are chamomile, marshmallow, alfalfa, meadowsweet, golden seal, and liquorice root.

• Glutamine is an amino acid that can reduce inflammation in the lining of the stomach and good results can be achieved by taking one teaspoon of pure glutamine powder twice daily in coconut, dairy or almond milk. For more information see page 31

• If you get an acute attack of heartburn it is effective to use an antacid preparation for quick relief. Avoid aluminium containing antacids; instead choose potassium or sodium bicarbonate, magnesium carbonate or hydroxide instead.

Gastritis

Gastritis is inflammation of the inner lining of the stomach.

Gastritis can be caused by:

• A poor diet high in sugar, refined carbohydrates or alcohol

• Chronic and repetitive vomiting due to many causes, including paralysis of the stomach (gastroparesis)

• The overuse of certain medications such as aspirin or other anti-inflammatory drugs

• Infection of the stomach with a bacteria called Helicobacter pylori (H. pylori). If this is not treated it can lead to peptic ulcers, and in some people, stomach cancer.

• Auto-immune inflammation of the stomach lining can damage the stomach so badly that it can no longer produce a naturally occurring substance (intrinsic factor) that is needed to absorb vitamin B12 from the small intestine. This causes pernicious anemia due to vitamin B 12 deficiency and can lead to disease of the spinal cord. It is always wise to check your blood levels of vitamin B 12, as if they are very low, you could have pernicious anemia due to autoimmune gastritis. Injections of vitamin B 12 must be given as it is not possible to absorb vitamin B 12 from the diet or from vitamin supplements. Vitamin B 12 injections can completely restore your health in such cases. It is important to avoid gluten in the diet if you have autoimmune gastritis and pernicious anemia.

- Bile reflux: A back flow of bile into the stomach from the duodenum. The bile tract (duct) empties bile into the duodenum to digest fats. Bile can be very irritating to the stomach and does not belong there. Bile reflux can be helped by improving your liver function with a good liver formula such as LivaTone Plus and a magnesium powder. Digestive enzymes taken at beginning of meals and Aloe Vera taken one hour after food can also provide relief.

Gastritis must be treated or it can lead to bleeding from the stomach and iron deficiency anemia. It may also increase the risk of developing stomach cancer.

Symptoms of gastritis vary and there may be no symptoms at all. The most common symptoms include:

- Nausea or vomiting

- Abdominal bloating

- Pain over the upper abdomen

- Indigestion or reflux and heartburn

- Burning or gnawing feeling in the stomach between meals or at night

- Hiccups

- Bad breath

- Loss of appetite

- Vomiting red blood or coffee ground-like material

- Black, tar like feces (caused by bleeding from the stomach)

Tests to Diagnose Gastritis

Visualization of the stomach and duodenum through an endoscope is required. An endoscope is a thin tube containing a tiny camera, which is inserted through your mouth and down into your stomach to look at the stomach lining. Through the endoscope a biopsy of the stomach lining (a tiny sample of tissue is removed) can be done.

This is sent to a laboratory for analysis to check for inflammation, cancer and infection. Blood tests are needed to check for liver function, anemia, iron and vitamin B 12 deficiencies and a breath test should be done to exclude infection with Helicobacter Pylori. A fecal occult blood test (stool test) can check for the presence of blood in your feces which can be a sign of gastritis.

Treatment for gastritis:

For gastritis caused by Helicobacter Pylori infection, a course of several antibiotics plus an acid blocking drug is prescribed for several weeks. Helicobacter Pylori is an opportunistic parasite, and will return if you go back to eating poorly. If you follow my suggestions for peptic ulcers and reflux on pages 72 to 77, this will generally heal the gastritis. Once the underlying cause is treated, the gastritis will be cured. In some cases drugs to reduce stomach acid will be prescribed – see page 74

You can also try a supplement containing hydrochloric acid in the form of betaine hydrochloride (HCL). This should be taken in the middle of meals and can be very effective.

Gastroparesis – slow stomach emptying

Gastroparesis is a condition in which there is delayed emptying of the stomach. Normally the stomach's muscles contract efficiently in order to propel food from the stomach into the small intestine. However if the muscles (or the nerves that control the muscles) are not working normally, food empties too slowly, or hardly at all, and remains in the stomach for way too long.

Most cases of gastroparesis have no obvious cause and are called idiopathic. Gastroparesis can also be caused by diseases of the nervous system, diabetes and some medications.

The muscles of the stomach are controlled by the vagus nerve and when they contract, food breaks up and moves through the gastrointestinal (GI) tract. Gastroparesis can occur when the vagus nerve is damaged by disorders of the nervous system, injury or diabetes and this causes the stomach muscles to have very weak or no contractions. Food then moves very slowly from the stomach to the small intestine or stops moving altogether. Other causes of gastroparesis include intestinal surgery and nervous system diseases such as Parkinson's disease or multiple sclerosis.

The much less common condition of rapid gastric emptying can cause diarrhea and episodes of weakness or light-headedness following meals. This is referred to as the "dumping" syndrome. Common causes of rapid gastric emptying include surgery of the stomach and diabetes mellitus.

What are the symptoms of gastroparesis?

The most common symptoms of gastroparesis are a feeling of fullness after eating only a small amount of food and nausea and vomiting up undigested food; this can sometimes happen several hours after a meal.

Other symptoms of gastroparesis may include:

- abdominal bloating
- weight loss
- lack of appetite
- gastro-esophageal reflux (GERD), also called acid reflux
- pain in the stomach area (upper central abdomen)

Symptoms may vary from mild to severe and gastroparesis can be hard to diagnose because people experience a range of symptoms similar to those of other diseases.

Gastroparesis is diagnosed through a thorough history, physical examination, blood tests and tests to rule out blockage or structural problems in the GI tract. The most important test is called a gastric emptying test.

Gastric emptying test. This test is called gastric scintigraphy. The patient is given a meal that contains a small amount of radioactive material. The rate of gastric emptying is measured at 1, 2, 3, and 4 hours after the meal. If more than 10 percent of the meal is still in the stomach at 4 hours, the diagnosis of gastroparesis is confirmed.

Other tests to exclude gastroparesis

- Upper gastrointestinal (GI) endoscopy. A gastroscope (a small, flexible tube with a light) is passed through the mouth to see the upper GI tract (the esophagus, stomach, and duodenum). The test may show blockage in the upper gastro-intestinal tract or large bezoars. Bezoars are solid collections of food, mucus and vegetable fiber that cannot be digested in the stomach.

• Upper GI X-ray series. This type of X-ray may be done to look at the shape of the small intestine. During this test the patient stands in front of an X-ray machine and drinks a chalky white radio-opaque liquid called barium. The barium coats the inside of the small intestine, making signs of gastroparesis show up more clearly. Gastroparesis is likely if the X- ray shows food in the stomach after fasting.

• Breath test. The patient eats a meal containing a small amount of radioactive material. After eating, samples of the breath are taken for several hours to measure the amount of radioactive material in the breath. The results determine how fast the stomach is emptying.

• Smart Pill. This pill is swallowed to record information that provides a detailed record of how quickly food travels through each part of the digestive tract.

Treatment of gastroparesis

Unfortunately for most patients treatment does not cure gastroparesis. This is because gastroparesis is usually a long-lasting and recurring condition. Patients learn to manage the symptoms so they can remain as comfortable and active as possible.

Eating small meals frequently is a must, as the sluggish stomach cannot cope with normal sized meals. If less food enters the stomach it does not become so full which enables it to empty more easily. Food must be chewed for longer and drinking fluids with food is not advised. After eating a meal you may find that going for a walk or sitting for 2 hours may assist with gastric emptying.

People with gastroparesis should minimize their intake of large portions of foods high in fiber or large pieces of meat because the undigested parts of the food may remain in the stomach too long. Sometimes, the undigested parts form bezoars.

A liquid or puréed diet may be best and healthy soups and smoothies can be made in a high powered blender such as a Thermomix or Vitamix. As liquids tend to empty more quickly from the stomach, many patients find a puréed diet reduces their symptoms.

When the most extreme cases of gastroparesis lead to severe vomiting and/or dehydration, intravenous (IV) fluids or IV nutrition can be given.

Medications

Several prescription medications are available to treat gastroparesis. Sometimes a combination of medications may be the most effective treatment.

Metoclopramide is a medication that stimulates stomach muscle contractions to speed up gastric emptying. Metoclopramide reduces nausea and vomiting and is taken 20 to 30 minutes before meals and at bedtime. Possible side effects of metoclopramide include fatigue, sleepiness, and depression. In rare cases it can cause an irreversible side effect on the nervous system called tardive dyskinesia, which affects movement.

Erythromycin is an antibiotic drug that can be used at low doses, to improve gastric emptying by increasing the contractions of the stomach. Possible side effects of erythromycin include nausea, vomiting, and abdominal cramps.

Botulinum Toxin is a nerve blocking chemical known as Botox. After passing an endoscope tube into the stomach Botox is injected into the Pylori (the opening from the stomach into the duodenum) to keep the Pylori open for longer periods of time to make it easier for the stomach to empty. Early research trials showed modest improvement in gastroparesis symptoms and the rate of gastric emptying following the Botox injections, but other studies have failed to show much long term improvement

Gastric Electrical Stimulation

This treatment may be effective for some people whose symptoms do not improve with dietary changes or medications. A gastric neuro-stimulator is a surgically implanted battery-operated device that sends mild electrical pulses to the stomach muscles to make the stomach muscles contract. Once implanted, the settings on the battery-operated device can be adjusted to determine the settings that best control symptoms.

Celiac Disease

Celiac disease is an autoimmune disease which damages the lining of the small intestine. It is caused by intolerance to gluten protein in the diet. Celiac disease can be hereditary so check your family history. Gluten is a protein found in the grains wheat, barley, rye and oats. The term "intolerance" is not the same as "allergy," and implies a more chronic or long term adverse reaction in the body.

The gluten damages the cells lining the small intestine, and the mucosal surface becomes flat, losing its normal folds (these folds are known as villi). These damaged mucosal cells are unable to absorb nutrients from the food and severe nutritional deficiencies eventually occur.

Celiac disease is common in Western nations with an incidence of approximately 1 in 100. The disease can begin at any age, and in children, it appears after weaning them onto gluten containing foods. In adults it usually begins in the third and fourth decade, and is more common in females.

The symptoms are usually very gradual in onset and may start with only fatigue. Common symptoms include abdominal discomfort, bloating, diarrhea and weight loss. There is difficulty in absorbing fat from ingested food, which causes the bowel actions to become large, pale and fatty; such stools tend to float on top of the water and are difficult to flush down the toilet.

Mouth ulcers, skin rashes and dermatitis around the corners of the mouth are common. Deficiencies of minerals (especially iron, zinc and selenium) and vitamin D are very common, as these things cannot be absorbed through the damaged intestinal lining. White spots in the nails can indicate zinc deficiency. People with celiac disease have a higher incidence of other autoimmune diseases (such as thyroid, diabetes type 1, inflammatory bowel disease and liver disease).

Many of the symptoms of celiac disease are similar to those of irritable bowel syndrome (IBS), so if symptoms do not abate with treatment for IBS, it is important to think of excluding celiac disease.

A blood test is available to detect this abnormal sensitivity to gluten. It is called the antigliaden antibody test. This test is more accurate in children, and in adults can give false results - either false positives or false negatives. You can also have a blood test to check if you have the genetic pattern that predisposes to gluten intolerance – this is called the HLA DQ Genotype test.

An accurate diagnosis of celiac disease is made by removing a tiny piece of the mucosal lining of the upper small intestine for examination under a microscope. This is called a biopsy and is done through a fiber optic telescope (gastroscope) passed through the mouth under an anesthetic.

Thankfully celiac disease responds extremely well to dietary modification. If patients stick to a gluten free diet they generally remain very well, and the mucosal lining of the small intestine returns to normal. Normal absorption of nutrients is then possible, although it is important to check periodically for deficiencies of iron, zinc, folic acid, vitamin B 12 and the fat-soluble vitamins (vitamins A, D, E and K). This is easily done with a blood test.

Because celiac patients are more likely to suffer with other types of immune dysfunction, I think it is wise for them to supplement their diets with Vitamins E, C, D, A and the minerals selenium and zinc. It is also important to boost the intake of omega 3 essential fatty acids by eating oily fish, chia seeds, walnuts, hemp seeds and ground flaxseeds.

If your diagnosis of celiac disease was delayed until later in life, the long term ingestion of gluten may have caused chronic damage to your small intestine and this may take several years to completely repair. I recommend that glutamine powder is taken in a dose of 2 to 5 grams twice daily in coconut or rice milk to speed up healing of the intestinal lining.

If you have had a delayed diagnosis, you probably have deficiencies of zinc, selenium, iron, calcium and the fat soluble vitamins (A, D, E and K). I highly recommend you supplement with these nutrients and take them individually, as the doses found in multivitamin and mineral tablets will be inadequate. Take fat soluble vitamins with food that contains fat. Check your finger nails for white spots and if you have a lot of these, this shows that you are mineral deficient. Ask your doctor to check your blood levels of vitamin B 12, and if these are deficient, you will benefit from a course of monthly injections of vitamin B 12.

A supplement of digestive enzymes will improve your absorption of essential nutrients.

Gluten Intolerance

In some people the protein gluten can cause a wide variety of health problems affecting the immune system. This is true even though they may NOT have or ever develop celiac disease. Yes that's correct - you can be intolerant to gluten even though you do NOT have celiac disease. Many doctors and patients do not understand this association, and because patients are told that they are not a celiac, they are told they can continue to eat gluten; unfortunately for them, their problems will remain, recur or become worse.

Risk factors or clues that you may be gluten intolerant include -

- If you have Crohn's Disease or Ulcerative Colitis

- If you have unexplained bowel problems for which a specialist doctor can find no cause

- If you have rheumatoid, psoriatic or other types of inflammatory arthritis

- If you have lupus and/or other connective tissue autoimmune disorders

- If you have autoimmune thyroid problems such as Hashimoto's Thyroiditis or Grave's Disease

- If you have recurrent or chronic inflammatory skin problems

- If you have autoimmune liver diseases such as Primary Biliary Cirrhosis, Sclerosing Cholangitis or autoimmune hepatitis

- If you have unexplained deficiencies of zinc, iron and/or other minerals in your body

- If you have premature or severe osteoporosis

- If you test positive for the HLA DQ genotype – a blood test

- If you have a family history of Celiac Disease, Crohn's Disease or Ulcerative Colitis

- If you have a family history of bowel cancer and/or polyps

The best way to test if you are gluten intolerant is to eliminate ALL gluten containing foods from your diet for 3 to 6 months and observe the difference in your health and your bowel function. You can follow a gluten elimination diet under the guidance of a practitioner and if you need help please email our naturopaths at ehelp@liverdoctor.com

You can also have a blood test to check if you have the genetic pattern that predisposes to gluten intolerance – this is called the HLA DQ Genotype test. If you test positive, you may find a large improvement in your health if you follow a gluten free diet. It can take 6 to 12 months before you can really judge the benefit of a gluten free diet, so you need to be strict and patient. The genotype test is not always positive in people who are gluten intolerant and this is why a gluten elimination diet may be the best way to discover if you are gluten intolerant. Gluten is found in wheat, rye, barley and oats and in many processed foods and bottled sauces.

In genetically predisposed people, dietary gluten can greatly aggravate many different types of autoimmune diseases, thyroid diseases, intestinal and digestive disorders and skin problems such as psoriasis or eczema. Once gluten is eliminated from the diet these problems will gradually improve and usually resolve, especially if nutritional deficiencies are corrected. For more information see the book titled *Gluten, is it making you sick or overweight?*

Gluten Free Diet

This involves the exclusion of the following grains: wheat, rye, barley and oats. All foods containing gluten - whether it be obvious, (e.g. bread, flour, pasta, pastry and most cereals) or hidden (e.g. most sausages, sauces and stock cubes) must be avoided.

Allowed Foods - Gluten-free (GF)

- Rice, tapioca, arrowroot, maize, millet, sago, buckwheat, amaranth, quinoa and teff

- Nuts, legumes and seeds

- Poultry, meat and seafood

- Eggs

- Dairy products

- Vegetables and fruits

- Gluten-free (GF) bread, GF pasta, GF biscuits and GF crackers

- GF flour made from such things as potato, hemp, chick peas, soy and rice

- GF bran made from such things as rice and soy

There are many gluten free products available today and mandatory labeling has made it so much easier to find gluten free foods than ever before.

But ALWAYS read the labels on any product first before purchasing.

There are numerous restaurants now that specialize in Gluten Free meals. Some pizza houses make gluten free pizzas if you request it. However if you have celiac disease then you may choose not to have the pizza where regular gluten pizzas are made, as there could be cross contamination of gluten particles from the pizza oven or the utensils. Always ask.

Foods to Avoid (gluten containing)

- Any foods containing wheat, rye, barley and oats – these grains and their flours are found in regular breads, cereals, crackers, biscuits, muffins, cakes, pizza, pastry and pasta

- Spelt

- Semolina

- Pies, pasties, most beefburgers, most sausages, many tinned meats

- Meat or fish with breadcrumbs or batter, fish cakes, Potato croquettes

- Barley water

- Beer

- Most stock cubes and gravy mixes

This list is not exhaustive and there are other things that you may need to avoid. This is because it is not always possible to tell from food labels if a processed product is gluten-free.

The Celiac Society produces complete lists of processed foods that are gluten free and if you would like more information contact the Celiac Society in your state.

www.celiac.org.au

www.glutenfreetraveller.com

Healthy Gluten Free Grains

Amaranth

Amaranth was the grain used traditionally by the Aztec Indians of North America. Amaranth is now becoming a popular again amongst health conscious people. It is very high in protein and is a good source of complex carbohydrates. Amaranth is gluten free and can be used as a substitute for wheat in those with celiac disease. It needs to be pre-soaked and cooked on a low heat to facilitate digestion. You can use it in casseroles and stews.

Quinoa

Quinoa is another ancient grain and was traditionally used by the Incas. It is high in protein and can be used as a substitute for rice and wheat in many dishes. It is easy to digest and those with wheat allergies or irritable bowel syndrome find it of benefit. Quinoa is gluten free and is tolerated by those with celiac disease. It is also good for those with intolerance to dairy products because it is very high in calcium.

Other gluten free grain substitutes – These include rice, teff, millet, buckwheat and yellow cornmeal. Teff and buckwheat should be tolerated by those with celiac disease. Millet is gluten free and can be consumed by those with celiac disease; however millet sometimes becomes contaminated with wheat and other sources of gluten during harvesting, storage and processing of mixed crops.

Note: Spelt is a form of wheat and contains gluten.

Amaranth Casserole Recipe

Serves 4

1 cup	Amaranth, cooked
1 cup	Rice or millet, cooked
3 cloves	Garlic
1 cup	Carrots, sliced
1 cup	Cabbage, chopped
1	Zucchini, chopped
1 cup	Capsicum chopped
1 cup	Fresh tomatoes, chopped
425g (15oz)	Whole tomatoes, tinned, chopped (keep juice)
4 tbsp	Olive Oil, cold pressed
3 tbsp	Fresh basil
2	Shallots, chopped
2	Brown onions, chopped

Sauté olive oil with garlic, shallots and onions. Add all vegetables and sauté for 4 minutes.

Add canned tomatoes and their juice, amaranth and rice (or millet).

Simmer for 10 minutes and season to taste with sea salt, tamari, GF soy sauce or vegetable seasoning.

Make sure the vegetables are still crisp and do not overcook.

Hemorrhoids

Hemorrhoids are dilated swollen veins that occur in the lower rectum and anal area. They can be considered as varicose veins in the lower bowel. Blood clots may form inside the hemorrhoids, which makes them hard, painful and swollen.

Symptoms can range from mild discomfort or pressure to extreme pain in the back passage and anus, making it impossible to sit down. Hemorrhoids may cause anal itching, a mucous discharge or bleeding, with bright red blood seen in the toilet bowl and/or on the toilet paper after wiping. Hemorrhoids should always be assessed by a doctor to exclude more sinister causes of bleeding from the bowels.

If possible, try to control hemorrhoids with natural therapies and diet because surgery may only be temporarily effective. Furthermore hemorrhoids often recur years after surgery.

The surgical techniques most commonly used today are cryotherapy (freezing of the hemorrhoid), or placing rubber bands around the neck of the hemorrhoids to strangle them.

The causes of hemorrhoids include –

- Chronic constipation
- Pregnancy
- Liver diseases or liver congestion
- Obesity
- Excessive alcohol intake
- Stress
- Lack of vitamin C

Strategies to overcome hemorrhoids -

• Increase fiber in the diet by eating raw vegetables and fruits, unprocessed raw muesli, chia seeds, hemp seeds and ground flaxseeds. FiberTone is an excellent gluten free fiber powder and contains ginger powder, slippery elm bark, soy fiber, rice bran, peppermint powder, beetroot powder, broccoli powder, carob powder, spinach powder and tomato powder.

• Drink plenty of fluids such as water, dandelion coffee, vegetable juices and herbal teas. The best herbal teas are horse chestnut and nettle. Dandelion coffee can also be beneficial.

• Drink organic apple cider vinegar in a dose of 2 tablespoons in a small glass of water with every meal. This helps to shrink the hemorrhoids as well as improve digestion.

• Take a powerful liver tonic containing milk thistle, antioxidants ,selenium, taurine, vitamin C, B vitamins, folate, zinc, green tea extract, and N-Acetyl-Cysteine (NAC) to support liver function. This is available combined together in one capsule called LivaTone Plus. A congested or fatty liver can lead to hemorrhoids.

• Take vitamin E 500 IU daily in the form of mixed tocopherols. Avocados are high in Vitamin E so try to eat them regularly.

• Take vitamin C in a dose of 1000 to 2000 mg daily. Rosehips and bioflavonoids can also help to heal hemorrhoids. Other sources of bioflavonoids include all citrus fruits and their white pith, buckwheat and berry fruits (especially red and black colored); these strengthen blood vessel walls.

• Take a good quality fish oil and/or consume fresh garlic or garlic tablets to keep the blood thinner, which reduces congestion in the veins. Serrapeptase is an enzyme, which is available in capsules, and if taken twice daily can thin the blood and reduce inflammation.

• Creams or suppositories can be applied to the hemorrhoids or inserted into the rectum. These typically contain local anesthetic/steroid drugs for quick short-term relief from the pain of hemorrhoids which are swollen or have blood clots in them. For long term treatment, use herbal creams/ointments containing the herbs witch hazel, calendula, golden seal and/or hypericum. Castor oil and zinc cream can also be soothing.

• Sit in a warm salt bath with 3 tablespoons of sea salt dissolved in the water. This will provide cleansing and soothing of the anal area. If you are plagued with recurrent hemorrhoids, consider installing a bidet.

• Regular exercise and the avoidance of prolonged standing or sitting are important. Avoid straining during bowel movements. When hemorrhoids are present, they often cause a full feeling, or what is referred to as a sense of incomplete evacuation, after a bowel action. This may cause you to strain and push to get the last bit of stool out, when in reality all the stool is gone. In this situation further straining will only push the hemorrhoids out, causing prolapsed hemorrhoids.

• Reduce stress, as this can bring on a hemorrhoid attack. Magnesium supplements can help to reduce stress and also reduce constipation. Magnesium powders are more effective than tablets in this regard.

Diverticulosis

Diverticulosis occurs when tiny defects in the muscle of the wall of the large intestine (colon) allow small pockets or pouches (diverticula) to develop gradually over many years. Diverticula are common in people over 50 years of age. Diverticulitis is infection and/or inflammation of these pouches. Together, these conditions are called diverticular disease.

Diverticula on the Sigmoid Colon

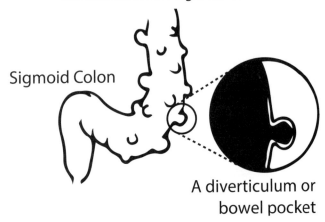

Sigmoid Colon

A diverticulum or bowel pocket

What are the causes of Diverticulosis ?

Lack of dietary fiber - In those who do not consume enough dietary fiber, the colonic muscles must work much harder to propel food along the colon to the rectum. These excessive contractions increase the pressure inside the colon leading to stretched and weakened areas in the bowel wall. The small pouches or diverticula then pop through or "blow out" in these weakened areas.

Excessive use of strong laxatives in those with chronic constipation can also cause diverticula, because these drugs lead to excessive colonic contractions and high internal bowel pressures.

Diverticulosis

There may not be any symptoms in some people whereas others will suffer with bloating, irregular bowel actions and some abdominal cramps and pain in the lower abdomen.

Sometimes undigested food can become trapped inside these bowel pockets, and then bacteria start to work on it, causing fermentation and putrefaction of the food particles. This can lead to foul smelling wind and abdominal swelling and cramps.

Many of these symptoms are similar to those of bowel cancer, and a specialist (either a bowel surgeon or a gastroenterologist) will need to assess these symptoms with a colonoscopy – your own doctor should refer you to such a specialist.

Diverticulitis

If the bowel pocket becomes very inflamed and/or infected, the condition of diverticulitis occurs. The bowel pocket may leak toxins and bacteria into the normally sterile abdominal cavity, which causes peritonitis. Symptoms of fever, nausea, vomiting and severe abdominal pain, particularly in the lower abdomen, may occur and admission to hospital becomes essential. Treatment with strong antibiotics, intravenous fluids and fasting is required. The diverticula pouches may rupture, spilling bacteria and feces into the abdominal cavity. This is a life threatening emergency, as it causes peritonitis and blood infection (septicaemia).

Complications of diverticulitis disease include:

• Rupture – a weakened pocket of bowel wall may perforate and the contents of the bowel can then escape into the normally sterile abdominal cavity. A perforated bowel is a medical emergency.

• Abscess – diverticulitis may lead to an abscess forming in the bowel pocket – this is an entrapped ball of pus.

• Peritonitis – this refers to infection of the membranes that line the abdominal cavity and envelope the abdominal organs. This complication is potentially life threatening.

• Bleeding – diverticula can start to bleed, leading to black or red colored stools. When bleeding occurs, it is important to see a specialist doctor to exclude other causes of bleeding.

How is the diagnosis of diverticular disease made?

Diverticulosis often exists for years without causing any symptoms and is often discovered during tests or examinations for other bowel conditions.

What tests are done to confirm the diagnosis of diverticular disease?

• A thorough physical examination – including a rectal examination

• A colonoscopy – a thin fiber optic flexible tube is inserted into the anus enabling the inspection of the entire length of the large intestine. This is done under a general anesthetic and is usually a day procedure.

• A Barium enema X-ray – a contrast dye is flushed into the rectum and colon via the anus and X-rays are taken to show the shape and size of the colon; this may show up pockets in the colon

• CT scan – this type of scan can detect abscesses within and outside the bowel lining

• Blood tests such as a full blood count, ESR and CRP – these should be done to check for signs of anemia, infection and inflammation

• Stool (feces) tests – these check for blood in the feces or the presence of unhealthy and dangerous bacteria.

Treatment of diverticulosis

The diet needs to be modified in those with diverticulosis.

• Do not eat foods containing small nuts and seeds, (found in some breads, muesli and cookies), as these small things can become trapped inside the bowel pockets. Seeds and nuts are very healthy and you may still enjoy them if you take the time to grind them into a fine powder in a coffee grinder or food processor. In this powder form they will not aggravate diverticulosis, and indeed should help the condition by boosting dietary fiber. Chia seeds can be well tolerated, and once they are softened by mixing with a liquid such as water or coconut milk, they can be very beneficial for the bowels. Eat them regularly and see the difference and you will be impressed. There is no need to grind chia seeds. There needs to be a gradual increase in dietary fiber. This will reduce the pressure inside the colon and improve bowel habits and reduce symptoms.

• Some sufferers find avoiding legumes (peas and beans), tomatoes and sweet corn also helps, and trial and error is required.

• FiberTone powder can be taken in a dose of 2 to 3 teaspoons daily to strengthen the bowel wall and reduce constipation.

• If enjoyed, animal meats can be eaten, but should be very fresh and very well cooked and eaten in small amounts only. Red meat is probably safer than chicken, as chicken can contain more bacteria, unless it is extremely fresh and very thoroughly cooked.

• Drink plenty of pure water in between your meals, as this will greatly reduce symptoms.

• Have smaller frequent meals with plenty of raw and cooked vegetables. Good fruits to eat are papaya, mangoes, pineapple, apples, pears, citrus and stone fruits.

• Take time in food preparation - this takes longer for those with diverticular disease because it is safer to eat your vegetables finely chopped or grated after they have been washed thoroughly. It is even better if you can afford to purchase a high powered food processor such as a Vitamix or Thermomix to blend whole fruits and vegetables into a whole-food soup. These machines can make green smoothies with things such as avocado, kale, carrot, mint, parsley, aloe vera leaves, apples and cucumber. You can also add glutamine powder to the smoothies for an extra healing and soothing effect. See page 51 for green smoothie recipe

• Herbal teas can help and the best ones are chamomile, dandelion, , ginger, peppermint, and golden seal, yellow dock and marshmallow. Do not sweeten with sugar – use honey or stevia or Nature Sweet Sugar Substitute

• Improve the amount of healthy bacteria in the colon by using a probiotic supplement – see page 26 and eating some fermented foods – see page 254

• Exercise regularly to encourage bowel function and peristalsis. Pilates and Yoga and excellent for improving the abdominal muscles

• Intermittent and short-term use of laxatives to treat and prevent constipation may be advised. See page 41 for the safest and most effective laxatives

• Colonic irrigations and enemas may help but can only be used if your own doctor agrees. They are safe in diverticulosis, but not in diverticulitis, when inflammation and the risk of bowel wall rupture are present

The long-term use of a mild antibiotic drug is often necessary to prevent further attacks if the patient does not want to change their diet or natural antibiotics do not work. See pages 24 and 25 for information on natural antibiotics for bowel infections

Surgery may be required to remove seriously affected bowel segments when symptoms are disabling and recurrent. This can be very effective, and indeed may be life saving, and should be done by a surgeon who specializes in large bowel surgery

Diverticulitis can be very serious, requiring immediate admission to hospital. Mild attacks can be treated at home with fasting, increased water and antibiotics but should always be assessed promptly by a doctor

Hospital treatment of diverticulitis may include:

- No eating or drinking – intravenous fluids are given to rest the bowel

- Intravenous antibiotic drugs

- Emergency surgery will be done if the pockets have ruptured or become obstructed. A colostomy may be needed if it isn't possible to rejoin the healthy sections of bowel and a colostomy bag will be fitted to the end of the healthy bowel. This is more common if the surgery is performed as an emergency. The use of a colostomy is generally temporary and the bowel can be rejoined after six to 12 months,

Bowel Polyps

Polyps are just a growth of tissue that develops on the inner lining of the intestine. A polyp can be raised and look like a pea on a stalk, or it can be flat.

Removing a bowel polyp through a colonoscope

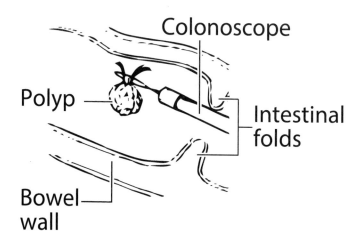

There can be just one polyp or multiple polyps. Most polyps are benign, but occasionally a polyp may develop into cancer. Not all bowel polyps are harmful, but some have the potential to develop into cancer if not monitored. Polyps tend to occur in the large intestine, called the colon; therefore they are commonly referred to as colonic polyps.

The discovery of polyps in your intestine should be taken seriously, because if dealt with promptly, you may be able to avoid the development of more serious bowel conditions.

There are 3 main types of colon polyps:

Ordinary polyps. These polyps commonly develop between the ages of 40 and 60. Most are not cancerous, but if not monitored, they could become cancerous in around 10 years. If members of your family have these polyps, you are more likely to develop them too.

Hereditary familial polyposis. This is a genetic condition where there can be hundreds or thousands of polyps in the colon. These polyps tend to grow very early in life, and they almost certainly become cancerous. Luckily the condition is not very common.

Hereditary non-polyposis colorectal cancer. This is also a genetic disorder but isn't as common as familial polyposis. Again, the risk of colon cancer is high. This condition is also referred to as Lynch Syndrome and close family members are also at heightened risk of breast and ovarian cancer.

What are the risk factors for developing bowel polyps?

- Being overweight
- Lack of physical exercise
- Advancing age, particularly over the age of 50
- History of constipation
- Having a family member who has had bowel polyps or bowel cancer
- Moderate to high alcohol intake
- Vitamin D and selenium deficiency, which are very common deficiencies

What are the symptoms of bowel polyps?

In most cases there are no symptoms at all, or the symptoms are so mild that they are ignored. A lot of people put up with disturbed digestive function their whole lives, and therefore don't notice the subtle symptoms of bowel polyps.

If there are symptoms, the most likely ones include:

- Constipation or diarrhea that lasts more than 7 days.

- Rectal bleeding and if you notice blood on the toilet paper after having a bowel motion, you should see your doctor. It might just be due to hemorrhoids, but it could be more serious.

- Unusually dark colored stools can mean blood in the stool and you should see your doctor.

How do doctors treat bowel polyps?

If your doctor has discovered polyps in your colon, several of them will be removed and viewed under a microscope. This is necessary in order to determine if they are cancerous. People with a history of polyps need to have regular colonoscopies to check the colon and see if the polyps regrow.

If you have had a bowel polyp, or a family member has had bowel polyps, it is vital to see your doctor regularly for a colonoscopy. If treated in the early stages, polyps are harmless and easily removed.

Strategies to prevent bowel polyps

- Eat lots of vegetables. Vegetables are an excellent source of fiber that is not harsh and scratchy to the bowel wall. Many people do not tolerate grains or legumes well, yet vegetables are easy to digest and they provide valuable bulk to the stool. It is very important to keep your bowel moving each day. Ideally you would have between one and three bowel motions each day. The longer the waste is allowed to stay in contact with your bowel wall, the greater the risk that polyps will form.

- If you struggle with constipation, you may need help from a gentle bulking and gluten free laxative like FiberTone. The ingredients in FiberTone help to sweep the colon clean and they are not habit forming. This is good because it means FiberTone will not weaken your bowel. Chia seeds are also excellent for those with constipation and should be eaten regularly.

• If you hold stress and tension in your bowel, and that results in constipation, magnesium powder can do wonders for this problem. It is very effective for people who get constipated when traveling, or while staying at someone else's home. Magnesium helps to relax and strengthen the nerves and muscles of the bowel.

• Try to avoid sitting for long periods of time. Many of us have a job where we must sit all day and that is unavoidable. Try to go for a walk before or after work, and try to make your weekends active. The exercise doesn't have to be strenuous; it just has to be regular. This will help all bowel problems.

• Try to drink between 8 and 10 glasses of water or herbal tea each day. That will have a cleansing effect on your bowel and soften your stool. You could put 2 tablespoons of chia seeds into a glass of water or milk and leave it to thicken for half an hour. Chia seeds are soothing to the bowel wall and they help to keep you feeling full and less likely to snack.

• Make sure you have optimal levels of vitamin D and selenium in your body. Vitamin D deficiency is incredibly common so it's best to see your doctor for a blood test. If you do not have time to get outside in the sunshine regularly, or you live in an area that doesn't receive much sun, you will need a vitamin D supplement – see page 106. It is also wise to take a selenium supplement in a dose of 150 to 200mcg daily because it has powerful anti-cancer effects. For more information see www.seleniumresearch.com

• Make sure you don't have elevated blood insulin levels. Insulin is a growth promoting hormone. It encourages more rapid growth of polyps, and also tumors, both benign and malignant. Having elevated blood insulin is also known as insulin resistance, metabolic syndrome, Syndrome X and pre-diabetes. The best way to lower insulin is to follow a low carbohydrate eating plan and exercise regularly.

Bowel Cancer

Cancer of the colon or rectum (known as Colo-Rectal Cancer or CRC) is a very common cancer affecting people in the Western world, with around 1 in 20 persons being affected. CRC is second only to lung cancer in terms of mortality rates. The incidence of CRC in Australia is one of the highest in the world and is higher again in New Zealand. The good news is that bowel cancer is one of the most curable types of cancer if it is diagnosed early before it has spread beyond the bowel. If this is the case the 5 year survival rate is 90%.

Risk Factors for Colo-Rectal Cancer (CRC)

1. Genetic factors - these are important and there is a genetic predisposition to bowel polyps and CRC. If a person has one first-degree relative with bowel polyps or CRC, their risk of CRC approximates to 1 in 8 over their lifetime. Spontaneous genetic mutations leading to cancer cells can also occur in bowel polyps in those with no family history of cancer

2. Dietary factors that can increase CRC, are a high sugar, low fiber, high alcohol diet. A high fiber diet reduces the usual risk of CRC by a whopping 50%

3. Inflammatory bowel diseases such as Crohn's Disease or Ulcerative Colitis - those with long-standing Ulcerative Colitis and Crohn's Disease are at higher risk of CRC

4. Aged over 50

5. A past history of bowel polyps

Signs of Bowel Cancer

Colo-Rectal Cancer (CRC) typically does not produce any symptoms or signs in its early stages and has often been growing slowly for years before it is diagnosed. Unfortunately often there are no symptoms or signs at all until the late stages of cancer growth.

When symptoms and signs begin they may consist of bleeding from the rectum, a change in bowel patterns (constipation, diarrhea, urgency), abdominal discomfort, iron deficiency anemia or weight loss. If you have any bleeding from the bowels, a gastroenterologist must do a colonoscopy. X rays such as barium enemas are not sufficiently accurate to investigate a possible bowel cancer.

Sometimes the cancer may spread to other parts of the body before it produces any symptoms. A common site of spread is to the liver and/or abdominal lymph nodes. Sometimes the bowel cancer is first detected when its satellite growths (metastases) cause enlargement of the liver and fluid in the abdomen.

Early Detection of Bowel Cancer

The chances of survival after CRC are related to the stage at which it is discovered. Early detection and treatment give a much better outlook. For this reason it is vital to identify patients in the early stages of CRC who will probably have no symptoms, as well as those with bowel polyps which may become malignant.

This requires screening of the general population and surveillance of high-risk patients.

Screening of the general population for bowel cancer:

- Ideally should start at age 50 and should be done every 2 years.

- Test stools for hidden blood (fecal occult blood test or FOBT). Although this is not 100% accurate, the FOBT is currently the most accepted and well researched screening test for bowel cancer. This is a free screening program provided by the federal government and you will be sent a FOBT kit in the mail. This includes an instruction sheet and equipment for collecting stool samples. Once completed you send it back to the nominated pathology laboratory and the results will be sent to you and your local doctor.

- If the FOBT is positive for blood, your local doctor will refer you to a gastroenterologist who will do a colonoscopy to exclude serious causes of blood in the stools.

Surveillance of high-risk individuals for bowel cancer:

- Ideally should start at age 40 with a colonoscopy to find polyps or early cancer.

- If no polyps are found, repeat colonoscopy every 3 to 5 years.

- If polyps are found they must be removed and colonoscopy should be done more frequently until polyps stop recurring.

Prevention of Bowel Cancer

- Have your blood Vitamin D levels checked and make sure that you are not low in this cancer preventing vitamin– see page 106

- Consume red meat only from grass fed animals – Australian lamb is generally healthy. In general consume red meat in moderation - say not more than 5 times per week.

- Reduce your consumption of preserved foods, especially preserved and smoked meats.

- Reduce your consumption of alcohol to no more than ten standard drinks per week.

- Increase your intake of omega 3 fatty acids from oily fish, chia seeds, hemp seeds, ground flaxseeds, free range eggs and walnuts.

- Eat plenty of fiber, which is found in vegetables, raw fruits, whole grains, cereals, muesli, legumes, seeds and nuts.

- Ensure an adequate intake of antioxidants especially vitamins C, A, E and selenium. Avocados are very high in vitamin E and are a super food for the bowels. I have met very few people with a perfect diet, and even if you do have one, in this day and age, you cannot guarantee that you will get all the antioxidants you need to reduce your risk of cancer. I highly recommend a selenium supplement in a dose of 150 to 200mcg daily to reduce your risk of bowel cancer.

- Look after your liver. A healthy liver will protect your immune system from overload. A strong immune system is your greatest weapon against bowel cancer.

If you have risk factors for gluten intolerance – see page 85, then avoid gluten as it may increase your risk of bowel polyps and bowel cancer.

You may be at risk from consuming gluten in your diet. The best way to test if you are gluten intolerant is to eliminate ALL gluten containing foods from your diet for 3 months and observe the difference in your health and your bowel function. You can have a blood test to check if you have the genetic pattern that predisposes to gluten intolerance – this is called the HLA DQ Genotype test. If you test positive you may find a large improvement in your health if you follow a gluten free diet. It can take 12 months before you can really judge the benefit of a gluten free diet so you need to be strict and patient. This genotype test is not always positive in all people who are gluten intolerant and this is why a gluten elimination diet may be the best way to discover if you are gluten intolerant.

How to increase your chances of survival if you have bowel cancer

• Consume easily digested foods such as vegetable soups, pureed vegetables and raw vegetable juices. Suitable juices are beetroot, carrot, mint, parsley, celery, apple, citrus, kale and cabbage. Do not overdo the amount of fruit and approximately 20% of the juice should be made from fruit and 80% from vegetables. The juices can be diluted with 50% water if desired. Drink around 500 to 1000mls of this juice mixture daily. Protein powder food supplements from whey, pea protein and glutamine are beneficial for those with weak digestion and poor appetite. These powders can be added to smoothies made with almond or coconut milk or sugar free Greek yogurt. Green smoothies are excellent and provide easily digested sources of cancer fighting nutrients – see page 51

• Eat fish at least three times a week, such as sardines, mackerel, trout, salmon and tuna (canned varieties are acceptable).

• Try to eat a wide variety of green leafy vegetables, raw and light-ly steamed. The cruciferous vegetables (broccoli, cauliflower, kale, Brussels sprouts and cabbage) have proven anti-cancer properties.

• Eat fermented foods – see page 254

• Take a probiotic supplement daily

- It is essential to take supplements of selenium 150 - 300mcg daily, and vitamin D 5,000 IU daily. You want your blood vitamin D levels to be at the upper limit of the normal range – see page 106

- Evidence from Japan suggests that an organic compound of germanium has anti-cancer effects. It appears to stimulate interferon synthesis and immune function. Germanium is present in garlic, shiitake mushrooms and champignon mushrooms.

- Eat Brazil nuts and garlic because they contain selenium, which has anti-cancer properties.

- To enhance digestion, eat foods that are rich in their own enzymes such as papaya, beetroot, sprouts, avocado, banana, mango and pineapple.

- Consume a low sugar diet as sugar feeds most types of cancer cells. Avoid all foods with added sugar. The only sugar that should be consumed is that found in fruit. Do not eat excessive amounts of fruit, as this provides too much sugar which can feed the growth of the cancer. The best fruits to consume are citrus, passion fruits and berries as they are lower in sugar. Cancer cells have a much higher requirement for glucose than healthy cells and cancer cells cannot grow without sugar. It is possible to starve cancer cells to death if you do not eat any sugar.

- Use foods and supplements to boost the body's production of natural interferon. Interferon is produced by normal body cells to keep cancer cells and viruses under control. It regulates immune cells and their defensive capability, and is vitally important for cancer sufferers.

The following substances will help to boost your natural interferon production:

- Chlorophyll (found in dark green vegetables)

- Vitamin C with bioflavonoids, 1000mg with every meal.

- Sea vegetables (such as hijiki, kombu, wakame, kelp, agar, Irish moss, nori, dulse)

- Blue-green algae such as Spirulina

Immune boosting herbs are:

St Mary's Thistle, Turmeric, Echinacea, Astragalus and Olive leaf extract.

Vitamin D is essential to fight cancer

Vitamin D supplementation has been associated with improved outcomes for immune disorders and cancer. Vitamin D deficiencies are linked to a higher risk of cancer, which is confirmed in over 200 epidemiological studies.

Vitamin D, which is made in large amounts in the skin when it is exposed to the sun, is actually a steroid hormone and not a vitamin.

Vitamin D can be found in such foods as oily fish, canned fish, cod liver oil, liver, eggs and full fat dairy products. It is also available in supplement form, with the current recommendation being that you take between 400 and 1000 IU of vitamin D 3 daily. Many people, especially those who avoid the sun or those living in cold countries, need much more than this and doses of around 5000 to 10,000 IU daily may be needed before you can get your blood levels of vitamin D into the higher desirable range. In people with a severe vitamin D deficiency, especially those living in cold climates or those with poor intestinal absorption of vitamin D, the use of vitamin D injections containing 600,000 IU, can be excellent and give a person all the vitamin D they need for 12 months.

Regardless of how you get it, make sure that you have an adequate amount of vitamin D in your body. It is easy to check your body's levels of vitamin D with a simple blood test; if your levels are below, or at the lower limit of the normal range, please take a vitamin D 3 supplement and get some sunshine on your skin. Recheck your blood levels after 3 months to ensure your vitamin D increases to the higher limit of the normal range. Make sure that you do not become deficient in vitamin D again.

Blood levels of vitamin D

The most important factor is your vitamin D serum level. It doesn't matter how much time you spend in the sun, or how much vitamin

D3 you take: if your serum level is low, then you're at an increased risk of cancer and osteoporosis. The only way to know your serum level is to have a blood test. It's recommended you check your level every three to six months, because it takes at least three months for it to stabilize after a change in sun exposure or supplement dose.

Vitamin D can be measured in two different units of measurement:

• In the USA the units used are ng/mL.

• In Australia and Canada the units of measurement are nmol/L.

The normal ranges of vitamin D for blood tests reported by different laboratories and countries vary significantly and you will be surprised by the large range between lower normal and upper normal – see table below

Lower Limit Vitamin D	Upper Limit Vitamin D
75 nmol/L	200 nmol/L
30 ng/mL	80 ng/mL

You don't want to be average here; you want to have levels of vitamin D that optimize your immune system to fight cancer. The optimal levels of vitamin D are higher than the average levels. I recommend you take enough supplements of vitamin D 3 and/or get enough sunshine to keep your serum vitamin D levels around 150 to 200 nmol/L or 70 to 80ng/mL.

Can Vitamin D become toxic?

The best way to optimize your vitamin D level is through sun exposure, but for some people this is not practical or possible, especially during the winter months. As a very general guide, you need to expose 40 to 50 percent of your entire skin to the sun for 20 minutes between the hours of 10 am and 2 pm; this is when the sun is at its zenith. There is no risk of vitamin D toxicity from ultraviolet B exposure.

Recent studies suggest that adults need around 3,000 to 8,000 IUs of vitamin D3 per day in order to get serum levels above 40ng/ml.

But this can vary a lot between individuals and the climate they live in. Even the conservative Institute of Medicine has concluded that taking up to 10,000 IU per day poses no risk for adverse effects.

Excess vitamin D intake can cause elevated blood calcium levels; so don't over dose on it - it's not a case of the more the better. Get your blood level checked every 6 months to find the dose of vitamin D 3 that keeps you in the optimal levels.

Apricot Kernels – can they help you to survive cancer?

Apricot kernels have been used as a "natural form of chemotherapy" and have been traditionally used in cancer patients who are looking for a nutritional approach to cancer treatment and prevention. The soft, bitter kernels are contained inside the hard apricot pits.

Bitter almonds or apricot kernels, contain Laetrile (also known as vitamin B17) in its natural state. The use of Laetrile as a drug was banned by the FDA in 1971 despite its proven benefits. However the source of Laetrile or B17, which are both the same, is legally available. Their natural source in apricot kernels is amygdalin, which some health authorities see as a serious cyanide poisoning threat.

How do the apricot kernels work?

Amygdalin contains different substances, namely glucose (sugar), benzaldehyde and cyanide. Cyanide and benzaldehyde are poisons if they exist as free molecules not bound to other molecules. Many healthy foods, including vitamin B12, contain cyanide and they are safe because the cyanide stays captured as part of another molecule.

Cancer cells are highly dependent upon sugar to survive and grow. The sugar in the apricot kernels surrounds cyanide. The cancer cell draws in the sugar, and when it uses the sugar, it releases the cyanide inside the cancer cell and only inside the cancer cell. It can be compared to a sort of smart bomb.

There is an enzyme called rhodanese in normal healthy cells, which traps some free cyanide and makes it safe by combining it with the mineral sulfur. Binding the cyanide to rhodanese converts it to a cyanate, which is a neutral non-toxic substance. Cyanate is easily excreted through the urine with no harmful effects to normal cells.

Amygdalin contains two glucose molecules and thus is attracted by sugar hungry cancer cells. A unique feature of cancer cells is that they contain an enzyme called beta-glucosidase that normal cells do not have. This enzyme unlocks the amygdalin molecules, which release the benzaldehyde and the cyanide, which is toxic to the cancer cells. Thus we could say that the cancer cell's beta-glucosidase enzyme causes cancer cells to self destruct by exposing themselves to the cyanide and benzaldehyde. This is how cancer cells are tricked and targeted by amygdalin. This is different to most types of chemotherapy, which does not discriminate and destroys healthy cells as well as cancer cells.

On March 10, 2010 an Australian mainstream newspaper told the story of a man who cured himself of cancer by consuming large amounts of apricot kernels while improving his overall diet. The article started with "Paul Reid should be dead. Diagnosed with a rare, incurable lymphoma, he was given five years, seven tops, by his oncologist." The article included a photo of a healthy Reid, smiling with a platter full of fresh foods at age 68, 13 years after his prognosis. (Sydney Morning Herald, source below)

As of that publication, Paul Reid was still on his organic diet, consuming apricot kernels daily for maintenance. His cancer curing protocol consisted of consuming 30 apricot kernels per day. Despite official warnings regarding cyanide poisoning from amygdalin, Reid did not suffer cyanide poisoning eating 30 kernels a day!

Cautions with apricot kernels.

The most important thing to fight cancer is your diet and there is no point taking supplements or apricot kernels if your diet is high in sugar and/or processed foods. Sugar must be avoided during any cancer treatment as it feeds the cancer cells. Sugar can allow cancer cells to thrive making them tolerant to amygdalin's toxic effects, so healthy cells have to cope with the burden of cyanide breakdowns from high amounts of amygdalin.

However some people consume too many apricot kernels and poison themselves, so doses need to be carefully controlled. You must follow the directions and do this under supervision from a health care practitioner. You can take too much of anything with an adverse outcome. Excess consumption of apricot kernels could leak some cyanide into healthy cells and cause side effects such as headaches, nausea or dizziness; this indicate it`s time to reduce the amygdalin dosage. Consuming sugar will make amygdalin more toxic and less effective.

The use of apricot kernels is controversial, as they have not been subjected to controlled clinical trials and many doctors think that their use is quackery or dangerous. But to completely negate the use of vitamin B17 on the grounds of toxicity is not logical, as all the drugs used currently in orthodox cancer therapy are extremely toxic.

Ref: Sydney Morning Herald article on Paul Reid`s remarkable recovery from cancer with apricot kernels http://www.smh.com.au/national/can-apricot-kernels-keep-cancer-at-bay...

How to get more amygdalin safely in your diet?

Consume the following foods and seeds-

- Kernels and seeds of fruit: The highest concentration of vitamin B-17 to be found in nature, after apricot kernels (bitter almonds), are the kernels and seeds in apples, cherries, nectarines, peaches, pears, plums and prunes.

- Legumes: Broad beans (Vicia faba), Lima beans, Burma beans, chickpeas, lentils and sprouted mung beans.

- Nuts: Bitter almonds, macadamias, cashews.

- Berries: most wild berries. Blackberry, chokeberry, Christmas berry, cranberry, elderberry, raspberry, strawberry.

- Seeds: Chia, flaxseed, sesame seeds.

Higher concentrations of B-17 are obtained by eating these natural foods in their raw or sprouting stage.

You can safely boost your intake of vitamin B-17 by:

Eating the whole fruit (seeds included), but not eating more of the seeds by themselves than you would be eating if you ate them in the whole fruit. Example: if you eat four apricots daily, the kernels in the four apricots provide adequate B-17. Another rule of thumb is to allow one fruit kernel (eg. peach or apricot) per 10 lbs of body weight, as a safe strategy in cancer prevention. You should seek advice from your health care practitioner as precise numbers can vary between individuals depending upon metabolism and dietary habits. A 150-lb woman, for example, might consume 15 apricot or peach kernels daily to receive a physiologically reasonable amount of Vitamin B-17. Too many kernels or seeds can be expected to produce unpleasant side effects and should be consumed in biologically safe quantities (no more than 20 kernels daily).

My Recovery from Bowel Cancer

A Case History by Trish Pemberton

It came out of the blue. I had always been healthy. One day when I stood up from the toilet I noticed a dark blood clot in the toilet bowl. I was puzzled. My first thought was 'maybe I've got hemorrhoids?' I didn't see this as a problem because there are treatments available to make hemorrhoids less painful, yet strangely, I didn't have any pain. I became concerned.

An ache in my heel had been a constant companion for more than a month. Massage didn't help. If I had known anything about reflexology before I was diagnosed, I may have been aware of what was happening inside. Later I found out that that part of the heel relates to the large bowel. When I woke up after my surgery I no longer had the ache in my foot.

I went to the doctor who checked me by probing in my anus with a rubber gloved finger. This was uncomfortable but not painful. The blood from hemorrhoids is light she told me. My clot was dark, I didn't have hemorrhoids. She considered my case urgent and that day made an appointment for me to see a surgeon. Everything happened so quickly I didn't have much time to think about what was going on in my body and what was going to happen. I went along for the ride as the doctors seemed to take over my life. I was in shock. I was so stunned that I didn't object to the suggested treatment. Apart from the blood clot and ache in my foot, I had no other symptoms.

There was no pain, no constipation or diarrhea. After I was diagnosed I was told by all and sundry, that I was too young in my early forties to have bowel cancer, especially as there is no family history of it.

The surgeon checked me using the same technique as the GP, but he probed further – it was quite painful. It proved that there was a mass close to the base of the large bowel. He arranged for me to see the doctor who performs colonoscopies. I was given instructions for the day before to take only fluids. From 3 pm I started to drink 3 liters of a dreadful mixture called Glycoprep, to prepare my bowel for the colonoscopy. It reacts with the bowel to clear it so that the bowel wall can be seen clearly during the process. About three hours later there was the first of many rushes to the toilet.

My Colonoscopy

At the hospital, dressed in an open-backed, neck to knee gown, I was wheeled to the operating theatre and sedated. I woke up in a screened area. The doctor confirmed that the mass in my bowel was cancer.

I went back to the surgeon to arrange the operation. He showed me a photograph taken during the colonoscopy. Whereas the bowel is normally round like a tube and clear, I had less than an eighth of the space open. The remainder was a cancerous tumor which had to be removed. I would need time in hospital to recover. It was like a bad dream.

The surgeon said that until he operated he would not know the extent of the tumor or how much of the bowel would need to be removed. He wanted to do the surgery in the morning because he liked to do the 'big jobs' in the morning. Small comfort! It didn't occur to me that I may die. I accepted that whatever the outcome, it would be right for me.

My Operation

The surgery was two weeks later. At 3 p.m. the day before the operation a nurse brought in the Glycoprep. Yuk! She commiserated with me about having to take the muck, but that was no help to me. She was not the one who had to swallow the stuff, I was!

On the morning of the operation the anesthetist gave me one of those fetching gowns to put on, checked my hands for a suitable vein, then put a needle into that vein. I thought I was being particularly brave!

I was given the pre-med injection through this needle instead of an injection in my backside. What a relief.

I have been told that the operation took 4 to 5 hours. When I was fully conscious the surgeon came to see me. He told me the surgery had been successful, that the cancer had been encapsulated and they had been able to remove the whole thing. It had not penetrated the bowel wall so I would not need chemotherapy or any further treatment. I was fortunate. I had a sense of relief, but I had not considered any other result. It was a process I had to experience for some reason or higher purpose.

During the operation they had attached a colostomy bag and a tube through a small hole in my side attached to a bag which seemed to have vacuum pressure to drain the wound. The colostomy meant I didn't have to ask for a pan or go to the toilet. I was on a drip and my body was functioning normally so there was waste to be removed.

When the drip was removed ten days after the operation I was given a medicine glass with 2 mls of water to drink every two hours while they checked my bowel function. The amount of water was gradually increased when it became obvious that my bowel was healing well. After this my diet varied a little - jelly and soup were added. Although I was not interested in food I realized I had to eat.

Once at home my appetite was poor for about a month. Tomato soup and toast were a major part of my diet for that time. To get back to eating normally took months. There are foods I cannot eat now that I used to enjoy and fatty things mostly make me feel ill.

Following the operation I had regular blood tests and check ups with the surgeon. Cancer cells show up in blood as an early warning. All the tests have been clear. I had the final check five years to the day from the surgery, but I have colonoscopies every three years as a preventive measure.

My Recovery

I went to a GP/Natural Therapist who suggested I increase my dosage of Vitamin C to help my body recover from the effects of surgery and to take selenium and vitamin D supplements. I also added a small handful of apricot kernels plus a probiotic supplement to help my digestion. I started eating more fish and took omega 3 oils and vitamin B12.

Bowel cancer does not strike only the elderly or those who have a family history of it. It can strike anyone at any age. I have a friend whose 17 year old daughter got bowel cancer. A major point to be recognized is that it may appear at any time in any person. It does not attack either sex in preference to the other, nor does it develop after a particular age, although I have been told that it is more prevalent in older people.

The way to recover from bowel cancer, is to catch it in time to conquer it and to take notice of every symptom. If, as happened to me, you pass a blood clot, have yourself checked. If, as happened to an older lady I know, you feel constipated all the time, or your bowel movements spurt, have yourself checked.

It is better to be safe than sorry. Your local GP can give a preliminary examination. I know it may seem embarrassing or uncomfortable to some people to discuss this area of their bodily functions but it is worth it. It really is worth it.

Talking to various people about my experience of the cancer and how it has affected my life, I am uncovering feelings of my early years. I have been told that the person developing cancer has been bottling up emotional pain over many years. A bad diet including a lot of refined foods, sugars and processed flours, may be a trigger for some illnesses. However, I don't think anyone has yet successfully explained how one gets cancer.

It is only now, five years down the track, and I realize that I went through a lot of experiences, both emotionally and physically. I have had to adjust to the physical problems caused by the bowel cancer, and to come to terms with my body being so damaged by the surgery to remove it. I had imagined the wound to be a long straight line. However, I did not realize just how long or how wide it was until I summoned up enough courage to look at it. It was as if not looking at it meant it didn't happen, that the surgeon had been able to operate so as not to damage the surface of the skin. I didn't take this idea much further. I carefully avoided looking at my stomach area.

There was a feeling of grief on first seeing the wound. It was a shock to see the damage to my body. The color of the scar has eased from angry dark red to a paler dark pink over the five years, but it and the staple marks are with me for the rest of my life. My scar is a reminder to me that we cannot take life for granted. I still look at it with amazement. It did happen to me. I went through major surgery for the removal of a cancerous growth. I would not have survived but for seeing that blood clot and doing something about it.

Thoughts that I may not have time later to do the things that I had been putting off, only came to me as I heard of people who had died from not having discovered their cancer early enough, or not taking note of the symptoms they were experiencing.

My feelings at discovering that I had bowel cancer and that I would have to be operated on were of total disbelief. For most of my life, anything negative that has happened to me, I suppressed. The cancer would not be suppressed - it wanted to be looked at. My belief now is that I went through the experience of having and recovering successfully from bowel cancer so that I am able to write about it from a positive viewpoint to help others.

Chapter 4

Digestive and Related Problems

Candida Overgrowth

Candidiasis is a fungal infection caused by yeasts that belong to the genus Candida. There are over 20 species of Candida yeasts that can cause infection in humans, the most common of which is Candida albicans. Candida yeasts may normally live on the skin and in some body cavities (such as the mouth, vagina, nose and intestines) without causing symptoms of infection or disease. However, if an overgrowth of these yeasts occurs, symptoms of infection may occur.

Candida fungi usually live harmlessly along with the "friendly" species of bacteria that colonize the gastrointestinal tract and the growth of candida is kept under control by a healthy immune system and the actions of the friendly bacteria in the gut. Candida fungi and other yeasts, can multiply out of control if the numbers of friendly bacteria in your gut are reduced. In those with a lowered resistance, caused by diseases such as AIDS, diabetes or cancer chemotherapy, severe candida infections may occur. Other causes of candida infection include a high sugar diet and excessive use of broad spectrum antibiotic drugs, immunosuppressant drugs or steroid drugs. In some women high doses of the female hormone estrogen found in some oral contraceptive pills or during pregnancy may cause an overgrowth of candida.

Symptoms of Candida

As the candida yeast flourishes in the intestines, the bowels become an overactive fermentation tank. This causes excessive gas and abdominal bloating. There may be a thick white vaginal discharge and itchy anus and vulva. The tongue may develop a thick white coating and white patches appear in the mouth. Candida often causes a rash in various moist folds of the skin such as under the breasts or in the armpits and I see this a lot in diabetics.

Candida albicans can change its form from a simple non- invasive cell to an invasive mycelial form which has tendrils (tentacles) - see following diagram.

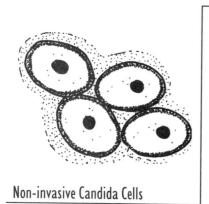

Non-invasive Candida Cells

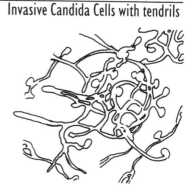

Invasive Candida Cells with tendrils

These tendrils grow like roots and can penetrate the wall of the bowel, and act like a leaking pipe through which waste products and toxins can enter directly into the bloodstream. This means that the toxins do not go directly to the liver which is thus unable to quickly break down these toxins; this can then cause symptoms such as fatigue, brain dysfunction, allergies and mysterious health problems.

A surprising case of intestinal yeast overgrowth in an adult male was reported in the Australian Doctor Magazine. The yeast overgrowth had followed a one month course of antibiotic drugs given to this man. Over the next several years this man was totally unaware that his bowels were overloaded with yeasts and the only symptoms he had was a foggy or muddled brain.

He told his doctor that he felt drunk so the doctor tested his blood alcohol level which was elevated. This perplexed him because in reality he rarely drank alcohol. His wife and doctor came to believe that he must be hiding an alcohol problem. He put up with this semi-drunken state of mind for several more months.

Finally he had a test to culture the types of bacteria and fungi in his stools – guess what was found? A very high concentration of the type of yeast that's used to brew beer! He was making alcohol inside his intestines and this was being absorbed into his blood stream. He was finally cured by a course of anti-fungal drugs.

This true case history is fascinating because it illustrates the profoundly adverse effect that antibiotic drugs can have on healthy gut bacteria and also how an overgrowth of unfriendly yeasts and bacteria in our intestines can seriously impair our mental state. It could be the reason we are mentally flat, depressed or have some cognitive impairment.

To test the types of bacteria and yeasts growing in your intestines have a stool microscopy and culture. For more information see pages 45 to 46.

Anti-Candida Diet

• Avoid yeast extracts such as vegemite and marmite, alcohol containing sugar (unsweetened spirits are generally safe), pickles and preserves containing sugar, jams, canned fruits, dried fruits, peanuts, melons and any fruit that is moldy. It is best to remove skin on all fruits if you have candida.

• Avoid bread, muffins, pastries, cakes, and biscuits and all foods containing white sugar, baker's yeast and flour. Avoid lollies, sugary sweet drinks, and any foods containing malt as an additive.

• Avoid every type of sugar, including raw brown sugar, molasses and honey, as they feed candida and other unhealthy yeasts in the bowel. It may be possible to use small amounts of a good quality honey (such as manuka honey) because honey contains natural antibiotics that stop fungi and bacteria from growing. It is trial and error but many people with severe yeast infections will need to avoid all sweeteners including honey. This can be hard if you are a honey lover! Stevia is not a problem for those with yeast infections. The sugar alcohols such as Xylitol, Maltitol and Erythritol are generally safe to use as they are not fermented by bacteria and yeasts. Thus the sugar like natural sweetener called Nature Sweet Sugar Substitute should be safe to use.

• Fruit can usually be eaten provided it is very fresh and free of moldy areas. Restrict the intake of fruits to no more than 2 pieces daily. In those with severe candida, fruit should be totally avoided for the first three months.

• Coconut milk or almond milk or A 2 dairy milk may be used; however, be sure to avoid brands that contain malt, sugar or maltodextrin.

• The diet should be high in fiber and healthy fats from seeds such as ground flaxseed, ground pumpkin seeds, chia seeds, hemp seeds, non-hulled tahini paste, avocados and coconut oil. Coconut oil is particularly effective against several intestinal parasites including Helicobacter Pylori bacteria and candida. Coconut oil contains lauric acid, which has infection fighting properties. You can cook or roast with coconut oil and also add it to smoothies or eat it off the spoon. Don't worry that it will make you put on weight, it will not and it has no effect on your cholesterol.

• Consume more raw and cooked vegetables as they are high in fiber. Fiber ensures that the contents of the bowel are emptied regularly which reduces the risk of candida building up in the bowel .

• Greek-style yogurt or coconut yogurt contains friendly lactobacillus bacteria, which help to fight candida and can be consumed regularly. Please avoid brands of yogurt that contain sugar or fruit. You should also take a daily probiotic supplement – see page 26.

• Foods that have natural antibiotic properties will fight candida effectively if they are eaten regularly. The best ones are raw garlic (finely chopped, grated or juiced), raw ginger, onions, leeks, and radishes, cruciferous vegetables (broccoli, Brussels sprouts, cauliflower, cabbage) and cinnamon. Fresh garden herbs can fight candida if they are eaten regularly - the best are thyme, oregano and rosemary.

• Virgin Coconut oil- this contains lauric, acid, caprylic, and caproic fatty acids - which are short- to medium-chained fatty acids that work on breaking down the outer wall of yeast cells. The oral dose of coconut oil is 1-3 tablespoons daily as a therapeutic dose to kill excessive yeast; you will need to start low and build up the dose.

- Generally speaking eating mushrooms is not a problem for people with candida and some species of mushrooms help to fight candida.

These are some of the beneficial mushrooms:

Ganoderma lucidum (Reishi), Grifola frondosa (Maitake), Lentinula edodes (Shiitake) and Trametes versicolor (Yun Zhi)

Supplements to fight candida and other yeast infections are:

- Minerals - selenium and zinc boost cellular immunity, which is important to overcome any fungal infections.

- Vitamin C supplements are essential to overcome candida.

- Herbs such as Golden Seal, Thyme, Pau D'Arco, and Olive Leaf; these are taken as liquid tinctures, teas or capsules. Aloe vera liquid helps to reduce yeast infections – see page 262

- Oregano oil – you can get capsules of oregano oil, which contain the active ingredient carvacrol. Generally one capsule of 45mg of the oil contains 32mg of canvacrol. Take one capsule with meals.

- Undecenoic acid has been found to be helpful in some people – each capsule contains 250mg and the dose is 5 capsules, 2 to 3 times daily - this seems a lot but if you have bad candida you will take it!

- Grapefruit Seed Extract (GSE) – take GSE between meals. The usual dose of grape seed extract is 75 -300 mg daily. Grape seed supplementation for up to 12 weeks is considered safe at recommended dosage on the packet. Side effects can include headache and sore throat. Higher risk for bruising or bleeding occurs if GSE is combined with blood-thinning drugs.

- Fungi inhabiting the mouth may be reduced by oral swishing with an anti-fungal solution made with Lugol's iodine, wild oregano oil, grapefruit seed extract and a few drops of tea tree oil. Gargle and swish around mouth for several minutes before bed, then spit it out.

Candida becomes a parasite once it exists in excess amounts in your body.

I recommend a formula called Intestinal Para-Clean which contains the following:

- Wormwood flower and leaf (Artemisia absinthium)100mg
- Black Walnut Green Hull (Juglaris nigra) 100mg
- Cloves (Syzygium aromaticum) 100mg
- Garlic (deodorized from Alium sativum) 50mg
- Butternut root bark (juglaris cinerea) 50mg
- Buckthorn bark (Rhamnus frangula) 50mg
- Pau D'Arco (Trabebuia heptaphylla Bark) 50mg

see www.liverdoctor.com

The recommended dose of Intestinal Para-Clean is one to two capsules with every meal. If you forget, just take them with a small amount of food. To eradicate candida, you may need to take them for 6 to 8 weeks. They are quite safe but do not take if pregnant or breastfeeding

Medical treatment of Candida

If rapid relief is required, or natural therapies are not powerful enough, you can ask your doctor for a script for a safe anti-fungal drug. The safest one is Mycostatin tablets or liquid, as it is not absorbed from the gut and works only in the intestines and mouth to kill the candida. This medication is very safe and non toxic.

Lufenuron

Lufenuron is an effective over the counter (OTC)/off-label anti-candida medicine. It is widely used by veterinarians. It works very well on all mammals with candida infections, although it is mainly used in animals. It works in humans but is not available in all countries and is not approved for human use by the FDA or TGA.

Lufenuron is well tolerated and safe and can be combined with other medicines. It does not damage beneficial gut flora.

Lufenuron destroys candida just as effectively as the oral drug Diflucan. It is a much safer drug than Diflucan because it does not damage the liver.

Lufenuron kills candida by making holes in its cell walls. Candida's cell wall is mostly made of extremely hard chitin. Humans do not need chitin in their body. Lufenuron destroys the chitin, which kills the candida by allowing the inside of the fungus to leak through holes in its cell walls.

If you want to try Lufenuron talk to your doctor first. If you have trouble getting Lufenuron it is sold at www.owndoc.com site. You will also find treatment details and results at this site. But tell your doctor first.

There are some types of anti-fungal drugs which are very liver toxic, and have been banned in some countries. So do not be too trusting and always check the side effects with the pharmacist before taking them. I do not recommend you take any anti-fungal drugs which have potential liver toxic effects.

Pancreas Problems

The pancreas is an organ that lies horizontally across the back of the upper abdomen behind the stomach.

The Pancreas

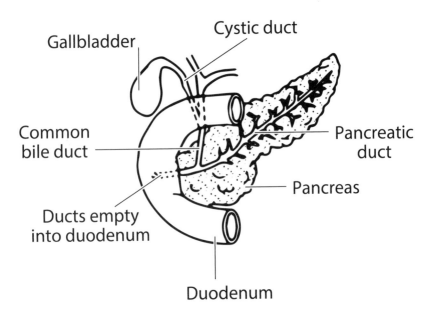

The pancreas manufactures the body's supply of insulin which controls blood sugar levels and fat metabolism. Insulin is released from the pancreas directly into the blood stream. Insulin blood levels rise after a meal, especially if it contains a lot of carbohydrate. If the insulin producing cells in the pancreas fail, diabetes will occur and insulin injections are required.

The pancreas also manufactures enzymes and secretes them into the pancreatic duct which empties into the small intestine to enable digestion of food. The enzymes produced by the pancreas include lipases that digest fat, proteases which digest proteins, and amylases which digest starch molecules.

Pancreatitis

The term pancreatitis refers to inflammation of the pancreas, and this may be sudden, severe and life threatening, or chronic and intermittent. Pancreatitis usually produces pain in the upper abdomen, which often spreads deeper into the back. The pain can vary from mild and grumbling, to sudden and excruciating, and is usually accompanied by nausea and vomiting.

The possible causes of pancreatitis are:

- Gallstones which become trapped in the pancreatic duct where it joins with the bile duct to empty into the small intestines. If the pancreatic duct becomes blocked, the pancreatic enzymes cannot flow into the intestines. In such cases the enzymes build up in the pancreas and digest the pancreas.

- Alcohol abuse

- Viral infections

- Poor blood supply to the pancreas

- Some drug side effects. A recent article in Diabetes Care 2013, 25th February on-line, brought to the attention of medical professionals "An increased risk of pancreatitis for patients with Type 2 diabetes on GLP-1 drugs. A US study in 2,600 patients with Type 2 diabetes who were hospitalized for acute pancreatitis showed exenatide (Byetta) and sitagliptin (Januvia) were associated with double the risk of acute pancreatitis compared with controls."

Sometimes the cause of pancreatitis is unknown and in such cases there may be hidden problems with the function of the liver and/or gallbladder, and in such cases the bile may contain excessive sludge and toxic waste products which inflame the pancreatic duct.

The pancreas can also become inflamed from being overworked in those who ingest too much deep fried food or refined sugars. This forces the pancreas to produce excessive amounts of digestive enzymes, and if the ducts within the pancreas are swollen or compressed with fat, these digestive enzymes can become trapped inside the pancreas and start to digest the pancreas itself. This process, known as auto-digestion of the pancreas, causes great pain, and damages the cells of the pancreas. This may result in cysts developing inside the pancreas.

Fatty Pancreas

Fatty infiltration of the pancreas is a benign (non-cancerous) condition and occurs when excess fat tissue has accumulated inside the pancreas. This fat tissue does not predispose to cancer of the pancreas. Fatty infiltration of the pancreas is more common in obesity, where fat gets laid down in other internal organs such as the liver. Severe fatty pancreas may be associated with chronic conditions that damage the pancreas. This is because, as the normal pancreas tissue dies off, it is replaced by fat.

The genetic disease of cystic fibrosis is another condition which damages the pancreas, leading to fat accumulation. It is important to check with your doctor if there is an underlying condition that has damaged the pancreas. If not, then you should try to reverse it.

A low carbohydrate diet should be followed and it is wise to avoid sugar and grains in the diet. Taking a good liver tonic and a supplement of N-Acetyl-Cysteine (NAC), 600mg three times daily, will assist to repair the pancreas. If you are overweight it is important to lose weight and this may reverse the fatty pancreas.

Fatty infiltration of the pancreas can be seen on an ultrasound scan or with other imaging techniques such as a CT scan or MRI.

A study published in the Journal of Clinical Endocrinology and Metabolism concluded that a new way to identify those at risk of becoming diabetic could be imaging tests such as ultrasound scans for fatty pancreas. Doctors at the University of Texas South Western Medical Center found that the accumulation of triglyceride fats in the pancreas was linked to a higher risk of diabetes and obesity.

Overweight subjects had about six times more pancreatic fat build up than subjects in the healthy weight range. Wow that's a huge increase! The diabetic subjects had significantly more pancreatic fat. The researchers found that the strongest predictor of excess pancreatic fat was the blood glucose level two hours after ingesting sugar.

If the body's usual storage site for fat - namely adipose tissue - gets overloaded by a high sugar diet, this causes the blood level of the fat triglycerides to rise. This excess triglyceride fat gets deposited in places it should not be, such as the pancreas, the liver and the heart.

The excess fat in the pancreas could very well be a cause, and not just a symptom, of impaired glucose tolerance in diabetics and pre-diabetics. Excess triglyceride fats stored in the pancreas release toxins, such as nitric oxide, which could damage the beta cells in the pancreas. The beta cells produce insulin, and if they are damaged too much, diabetes can occur.

Research is continuing to see if reducing pancreatic fat will improve blood sugar levels in diabetics. They want to test if pioglitazone, (an FDA-approved drug for treating diabetes that's known to break down excess fat in the liver), might owe its benefits for diabetics to its fat-fighting properties.

I personally think it is much safer to improve the function of the pancreas and liver with a low carbohydrate eating plan and a good liver formula plus supplements of NAC and selenium.

Pancreatic problems can be helped a lot by the following:

- Eat smaller meals and begin the meal with a salad.

- Follow a diet low in carbohydrates – this means you need to reduce sugar, processed breakfast cereals, bread, pastries, pasta, muffins, biscuits and cakes and anything which contains flour or sugar.

- Avoid excess alcohol and stick to no more than one standard alcoholic drink a day

- Avoid deep fried foods and trans-fats found in processed packaged foods.

- Avoid unnecessary drugs and painkillers

- Take vitamin C 1,000mg daily to reduce inflammation

- Take a good liver tonic containing milk thistle, antioxidants, selenium, taurine, vitamins C and B, folinic acid, zinc, green tea extract and N-Acetyl-Cysteine (NAC).

- Take a supplement of N-Acetyl Cysteine (NAC) to increase glutathione production, as this will help to reduce inflammation in the pancreas. The dose of NAC is one 600mg capsule, three times daily. Combine NAC with a supplement of selenium in a dose of 150 to 300 mcg daily, as this will boost glutathione levels which has a huge anti-inflammatory effect.

- Start to drink raw juices – good things to juice are citrus fruits, apple, carrot, cabbage, kale, ginger, celery, mint and parsley. Drink 200 to 300mls of raw juice twice daily. Make the juice fresh everyday or make a week's supply of juice and freeze it in glass jars immediately after making it. Note that bottled or canned juices will not have the same beneficial effect. Avoid bottled fruit juices as they are too high in sugar.

- Digestive enzymes should be taken with every meal, as the pancreas is probably not producing adequate amounts of its own digestive enzymes. If you do not take digestive enzymes you may develop malnutrition and digestive disorders, such as bloating after a meal.

There are vegetarian enzymes available for vegans and these are derived from plants.

The most potent digestive enzyme supplements contain an extract of animal pancreas and these are available with and without a script.

The higher dose animal-derived pancreatic enzymes may require a doctor's prescription. Creon is a pancreatic enzyme preparation available on prescription and is government subsidized for some conditions such as cystic fibrosis. Creon contains pancrelipase, which is an extract derived from porcine pancreas. Pancrelipase contains multiple enzyme classes, including lipases (to digest fat), proteases (to digest protein) and amylases (to digest carbohydrates).

Super Digestive Enzymes Plus formula contains a full range of pancreatic enzymes plus oxbile plus betaine hydrochloride. Available on-line at liverdoctor.com

What are the possible side effects of digestive enzymes?

Side effects are not common and generally people with poor digestion feel much better when taking animal pancreas extracts.

If side effects occur they can include:

- Nausea, reflux and/or mild stomach pain

- Change of bowel actions and rectal irritation

- Allergic reactions

These side effects can often be avoided by taking the enzymes in the middle of the meal or by reducing the dose of the enzymes.

Chapter 5

Food Allergies and Intolerances

Some people have multiple food and chemical sensitivities, which makes it difficult for them to follow a normal well balanced diet. These problems can be inherited (genetic) and can start at any age. They are often associated with a reduced ability of the liver to breakdown chemicals and proteins (antigens) in its detoxification pathways. Therefore it is always necessary to improve liver function in such cases, and this will gradually reduce the unpleasant reactions to foods and chemicals suffered by these patients.

The condition of leaky gut and unbalanced bacterial populations in the intestines is often present in sufferers of food and chemical allergies and this must be corrected.

It is worthwhile to source a reliable supplier of organically produced meats, fruits and vegetables so you can reduce your consumption of pesticides.

Use a high quality water purifier or drink rain water to reduce chemicals from your water.

You may find that foods high in natural sulfur compounds, which support the liver's detoxification pathways, help you. Foods high in sulfur include garlic, onions, leeks, radishes, cruciferous vegetables (broccoli, cabbage, Brussels sprouts and cauliflower), broccoli sprouts (available in powder or capsules) and eggs. If you are allergic to any of these foods, they should be replaced with other foods high in sulfur to which you are not allergic.

The adrenal glands also need to be supported in cases of severe chemical and food sensitivity, as they may not be producing sufficient steroid hormones such as cortisol, and this will increase the severity of allergic reactions. It is easy to test the levels of cortisol with a morning blood test. The adrenal glands can be helped with supplemental vitamin C and vitamin D. Essential fatty acids obtained from foods such as fish oil, oily fish, algae, chia seeds and ground flaxseeds can help to boost adrenal gland function

Vitamin B 5, also known as pantothenic acid, can strengthen the adrenal glands, and the dose required is 100 mg three times daily.

Food allergies are also often triggered when only partially digested foods are absorbed from the intestines, which may occur in those with an inflamed lining of the small and/or large intestine; this is also known as "leaky gut syndrome."

The liver finds it much harder to breakdown the larger proteins in only partially digested foods; this will overload the liver and can cause food intolerances. In this situation it is vital to take digestive enzymes in the middle of eating your meals. Pancreatic enzymes are available in tablet and powder form, and contain the full complement of digestive enzymes to break down food particles into smaller more easily absorbed molecules. You may need to adjust the dosage of the digestive enzymes under the supervision of your practitioner, as some people require much higher doses than others.

It is essential that patients with severe food and/or chemical intolerances consult a specialist in allergies who will perform extensive tests to accurately determine the things that must be avoided. The most common foods to cause allergies are dairy products, gluten, shellfish and peanuts. Artificial sweeteners, preservatives and food additives, can build up in the body, eventually causing allergic reactions. The most common offenders are MSG (monosodium glutamate), aspartame, sulphites, benzoates and nitrites, and artificial colorings. Check labels to see if these things are present and if so, avoid them.

Laboratory tests can be done through your doctor to check for food allergies. The most reliable test uses a blood sample to measure antibodies (such as IgG) that your body may be making against foods to which you are allergic. It is possible to test your reaction to many different foods using this IgG food panel test.

Those with severe manifestations of allergies such as asthma, swelling of the lips and throat or large hives, as well as patients taking cortisone drugs (steroids), can suffer fatal reactions to chemicals, foods and insect bites. These people should remain under the supervision of their doctor, and carry a syringe of adrenalin (EpiPen) for self-injection should an anaphylactic reaction occur and immediate help is unavailable.

Supplements that may help to reduce food and chemical allergies include:

A liver tonic containing milk thistle, antioxidants, selenium, taurine, vitamin C, B vitamins, folate, zinc, green tea extract and N-Acetyl-Cysteine (NAC) can improve the detoxification pathways in the liver, which enables the liver to breakdown offending substances such as amines, salicylates and other chemicals.

Extra taurine may be needed in a dose of 1000mg three times daily with meals

Vitamin C 1000mg twice daily to support liver and adrenal function

N – Acetyl – Cysteine (NAC) in a dose of 600mg capsules (take 2 to 4 daily until benefit is seen). NAC increases the production of glutathione in the liver. Glutathione reduces the production of free radicals which occur in excessive amounts during allergic reactions.

Selenium is vital for glutathione to function efficiently to protect you. Some people need higher doses of selenium (150 - 400mcg daily) to get a good improvement.

Glutamine powder can be taken in a dose of 2 to 5 grams, twice daily; mix it in juice or milk which is at a cool temperature. Glutamine is deactivated by heat. Glutamine repairs a leaky gut and supports the detoxification pathways in the liver.

Probiotics have been proven to reduce food allergies and chemical sensitivities.

Note: If you have severe allergies check with your doctor before taking any supplements.

The Royal Prince Alfred Hospital in Sydney has an excellent Food Intolerance and Allergy Unit to which you can be referred by your doctor. They also publish excellent books on food allergies and intolerances.

www.sswahs.nsw.gov.au/rpa/allergy/resources/foodintol/ffintro.html

Allergy Substitutes

Food	Substitute
Cow's Milk	Soy, Rice, Almond, Coconut and Oat Milk
Butter	Tahini, Hummus, Pesto (cheese free), Nut Spreads, Honey, Tomato Paste, Miso, Avocado, Olive paste
Cheese	Soy Cheese - grill or grate Avocado
Yogurt	Soy Yogurt or Coconut Milk Yogurt (Coyo is a known brand of coconut milk yogurt or you could make your own, see recipes on the Internet)
Ice Cream, Cream	Fruit Sorbet, Fruit Ice blocks, Lactose free cream, Soy Ice cream, Coconut ice cream or make your own using soy milk, rice milk or coconut cream. (Recipes can be found on the Internet)
Chocolate	Carob, Halva
Wheat	Rice, Corn, Quinoa, Buckwheat, Teff and pastas made from Soy, Millet, flaxseed, Cornmeal, Amaranth, Lentils

Self Test For Food Allergies

This involves measuring your pulse rate after eating the suspected food.

Measure your pulse rate at your wrist while you are sitting in a relaxed state before eating. Normally the resting pulse rate will be between 55 to 75 beats per minute.

Then consume the food that you think you may be allergic to and stay seated and relaxed. After 20 minutes measure your pulse rate again at the wrist. If your pulse rate has increased by more than 10 beats per minute (ie. gone from 60 to 72 beats per minute), you are probably intolerant to this food. This is all the more likely if you feel unwell, dizzy or nauseated as your pulse rate increases. Omit this food from your diet for 8 weeks and see if your health improves. You can then retest yourself with this food again and see if the adverse reaction persists. If it persists then permanently omit this food from your diet.

Are dairy products healthy?

This is a very individual matter as some people can eat dairy with no ill effects whilst others find that dairy products cause unpleasant symptoms such as respiratory mucous, sinusitis, bronchitis, constipation, diarrhea or asthma. In some people dairy products can upset the gallbladder. Thus trial and error is required.

If you are lactose intolerant you will find that dairy products cause diarrhea and bloating, unless you purchase the lactose free varieties.

If you have an autoimmune disease, I think it's best to keep your dairy intake controlled so that you do not eat large amounts at one time, and do not eat dairy products every day.

The healthiest dairy food choices are plain or Greek yogurt and pure cheeses (as opposed to cheeses processed with vegetable fats). White cheeses are easier to digest than hard yellow cheeses.

If you do drink cow's milk, I think that you need to be very selective, as not all types of cow's milk are healthy. It is becoming increasingly difficult for food and public health professionals to ignore the topic of A2 versus A1 milk. A1 milk has now been implicated in the genesis of Type I diabetes, heart disease, and allergies.

A2 milk is pure natural dairy milk and is free of permeate and additives. In contrast most dairy milk available today contains 2 main types of beta-casein protein, namely A2 and A1. Originally all dairy cows produced milk containing only the A2 type of beta-casein protein. A2 milk comes from cows specially selected to produce A2 beta-casein protein rather than A1. A2 milk is rich in A2 beta-casein protein and some people find that it assists their digestion.

Bowel Problems caused by FODMAPs

What are FODMAPS?

The term FODMAPS stands for **Fermentable Oligosaccharides, Disaccharides, Monosaccharides and Polyols** (FODMAPs). I can hear you saying – wow what a mouthful!

FODMAPs are sugars that exist in many different types of foods. FODMAPs exist in some dairy products, fruits and vegetables and grains.

FODMAPS can cause problems in some people because they are poorly absorbed from the small intestine, and when they arrive in the large intestine (colon) they can produce excess gas.

Studies have shown that eating FODMAPs causes irritable bowel syndrome (IBS) in some people. When people with IBS reduce or eliminate FODMAPs, their IBS often improves dramatically.

FODMAPs attract or draw water into the bowel and this results in increased flow of water through the bowel.

Because FODMAPs are poorly absorbed from the small intestine they travel to the large intestine where they are fermented by bacteria which produces gas. This gas production may cause excess wind (flatulence), abdominal bloating, cramps and pain. This may also cause diarrhea, which can be sudden and explosive. This may alternate with constipation.

FODMAPs are poorly absorbed in all people and this is normal. However those with a sensitive digestive tract or IBS may get symptoms if they eat FODMAPS.

FODMAPs are found in many foods we commonly eat and is an acronym for:

Fermentable

Oligosaccharides	- Fructans and galacto-oligosaccharides (GOS)
Disaccharides	- Lactose, sucrose and maltose
Monosaccharides	- Fructose, glucose, galactose
And	
Polyols	- Sorbitol, Mannitol, Maltitol, Xylitol and Isomalt

FODMAPs can be classified into two groups:

- FODMAPs that are partly absorbed (fructose, lactose, polyols)
- FODMAPs that are not absorbed in all people (fructans and GOS)

How do we diagnose dietary intolerance to FODMAPS?

Hydrogen/methane breath-testing is a useful method to identify if a person absorbs fructose, lactose and sorbitol effectively.

If breath tests are not available, a diet which avoids FODMAPs can prove if they are causing unpleasant bowel symptoms such as bloating, flatulence and diarrhea.

How do I follow the Low FODMAP Diet?

It is really a good idea to see a dietitian or nutritionist who has an interest in FODMAPS as you will need guidance. If you have bowel symptoms which interfere with your life it will be well worth the expense. They will teach you the ins and outs of a low FODMAP diet and how to maintain a low FODMAP pantry.

It can be quite complicated as when reducing FODMAPs in the diet, you need to maintain a healthy and well balanced diet

Low FODMAP food tips

- Choose gluten free and soy free flours and breads.

- Dairy foods should be low in lactose such as ripened cheeses (including Swiss and Parmesan). Choose lactose-free yogurt and lactose-free kefir milk.

- Select a variety of fish, meats and poultry that are FODMAP-free.

- Select nuts and seeds low in FODMAPs such as pecans, walnuts, almonds, peanuts, pine nuts, macadamia nuts and sesame seeds.

- Select fruits low in FODMAPs such as strawberries, bananas, blueberries, grapes, rockmelon, pineapple, oranges and kiwi-fruit.

- Select vegetables low in FODMAPs such as spinach, carrots, capsicum, eggplant, bok choy, tomatoes, zucchini and potatoes.

What are some of the challenges while following a Low FODMAP Diet?

The Low FODMAP Diet can provide adequate nutrition with careful planning. Your dietitian or nutritionist can ensure that high FODMAP foods are replaced with healthy and delicious alternatives.

If you are lactose intolerant, you need to ensure you obtain adequate calcium and vitamin D by consuming lactose-free milk and low lactose cheeses such as cheddar, feta, Swiss and mozzarella. Calcium enriched rice milk, spinach, tahini paste and canned tuna and salmon are high in calcium. You can also take supplements of calcium and vitamin D.

The low FODMAP diet is generally recommended for 8 weeks to judge its effect on your bowel function. After this time you should be reassessed by your dietitian who will gradually re-introduce some FODMAP foods into your diet.

Over time most people can relax their diet and may only need to avoid large amounts of some high FODMAP foods.

Table 1: Foods high in FODMAPs

Polyols	GOS	Lactose	Excess fructose	Fructans
Apples	Chickpeas	Custard	Apples	Artichoke
Apricots	Beans (e.g. baked beans, kidney beans, borlotti beans)	Condensed Milk	Corn syrup solids	Asparagus
Avocado	Lentils	Dairy desserts	High – fructose corn syrup	Beetroot
Cherries		Evaporated milk	Honey	Chicory
Isomalt (953)		Ice cream	Mango	Dandelion leaves
Longon		Milk	Pear	Garlic
Lychee		Milk powder	Watermelon	Leek
Maltitol (965)		Unripened cheeses (e.g. ricotta, cottage, cream, mascarpone)		Lettuce
Mannitol (421)		Yogurt		Onion
Mushrooms				Onion powder
Nectarines				Spring onion (white part)
Pears				Rye
Plums				Wheat
Prunes				
Sorbitol (420)				
Xylitol (967)				

Foods Low in FODMAPs

Fruits:

Banana, blueberry, boysenberry, cantaloupe, cranberry, durian, grape, grapefruit, honeydew melon, kiwifruit, lemon, lime, mandarin, orange, passion-fruit, paw-paw, raspberry, rhubarb, rockmelon, star anise, strawberry, tangelo.

Note: If fruit is desired, eat only small quantities.

Vegetables:

Alfalfa, artichoke, bamboo shoots, bok choy, carrot, celery, choko, choy sum, endive, ginger, green beans, lettuce, olives, parsnip, potato, pumpkin, red capsicum (bell pepper), silver beet, spinach, summer squash (yellow), swede, sweet potato, taro, tomato, turnip, yam, zucchini.

Cereals:

Gluten-free bread or cereal products

Buckwheat, amaranth

Rice, polenta, arrowroot, millet, quinoa, sorghum, tapioca

Milk:

Lactose-free milk, rice milk (check for additives)

Cheese:

Hard cheeses, Brie and Camembert

Yogurt:

Lactose-free varieties

Ice-Cream Substitutes:

Gelati, sorbet

Butter Substitutes:

Olive oil

Sweeteners:

Sugar (sucrose), glucose, artificial sweeteners – not ending in "-ol".

Honey substitutes like golden syrup and maple syrup (small quantities), molasses and treacle

Foods High in FODMAPs

Avoid these foods

Fructose

Fruits: Apple, mango, nashi pear, tinned fruit in natural juice, watermelon

Sweeteners: Fructose or high fructose corn syrup.

Large total fructose dose: Concentrated fruit sources, large serves of fruits, dried fruits and fruit juices, honey, corn syrup and fruisana

Lactose

Milk: Milk from cows, goats or sheep, custard, ice-cream and yogurt

Cheeses: Soft unripened cheeses e.g. Cottage, cream, mascarpone and ricotta

Fructans

Vegetables: Asparagus, beetroot, broccoli, Brussels sprouts, cabbage, eggplant, fennel, garlic, leek, okra, onion (all types), and shallots

Cereals: Wheat, barley and rye (in large amounts) e.g. bread, crackers, cookies, couscous, pasta and pastry

Fruit: Custard apple, persimmon, watermelon

Miscellaneous: Chicory, dandelion and inulin

Galactans

Legumes: Baked beans, chickpeas, kidney beans, soybeans and lentils

Polyols

Fruit: Apple, apricot, avocado, blackberry, cherry, lychee, nashi, nectarine, peach, pear, plum, prune and watermelon

Vegetables: Cauliflower, green capsicum (bell pepper), mushroom and sweet corn

Sweeteners: Sorbitol (420), Mannitol (421), Isomalt (953), Maltitol (965) and Xylitol (967)

Salicylate Intolerance

Salicylates are "aspirin-like substances" that exist naturally in plants and herbs. Some people have an intolerance to salicylates which causes unpleasant symptoms. Salicylate intolerance is worse in those with sluggish liver detoxification function or those with leaky gut. Salicylate intolerance can cause many symptoms from hives, hay fever, asthma, skin rashes, skin itching, cystitis and headaches to irritable bowel syndrome.

If you suspect that you have a salicylate intolerance consult an allergy specialist to confirm this, or follow a low salicylate diet for 8 weeks and see if your symptoms resolve.

Salicylate intolerance can gradually be overcome by improving your liver function through correct diet and perhaps a detox – see page 251

Supplements that may gradually overcome a salicylate intolerance include:

- Taurine - 1000mg three times daily
- Selenium - 150 to 300mcg daily
- N-acetyl- cysteine (NAC) - 600mg three times daily

These supplements will improve the phase one and two detoxification pathways in the liver which break down salicylates and other chemicals such as amines, drugs and caffeine.

If you are allergic to salicylates the table on pages 140 to 142, will help you to choose low salicylate food alternatives, which can be substituted in the recipes. You can flavor and season the recipes with the herbs that are low in salicylates. You will note from the table that garlic is low in salicylates. Garlic is a very good food to eat for those wanting to overcome a salicylate allergy/intolerance. This is because garlic is high in the mineral sulfur which supports the detoxification pathways in the liver.

You may be aware that many older people with vascular problems take low dose aspirin tablets to thin the blood. Aspirin is a synthetic salicylate. All salicylates thin the blood by reducing platelet stickiness, which reduces the tendency to form blood clots. By eating foods high in salicylates, (such as cayenne, curry, paprika, turmeric, cumin, mustard, ginger, tomatoes, radish, olives, capsicum and hot peppers), it is also possible to keep the blood thinner; this reduces the tendency to form unwanted blood clots in people with cardiovascular disease.

See the following tables for a list of foods high in salicylates.

For people who do not have salicylate intolerance, foods high in salicylates are extremely beneficial for the health of the cardiovascular system.

Food Salicylate Content Table

Fruits NEGLIGIBLE	LOW	MODERATE	HIGH	VERY HIGH
Pear (peeled)	Paw-paw Golden & delicious apple	Pear (with peel) Loquat Custard apple Red Delicious apple Persimmon Lemon Fig Rhubarb Mango Tamarillo	Passion-fruit Mulberry Tangello Grapefruit Avocado Peach Mandarin Granny Smith apple Nectarine Watermelon Lychee Jonathan apple	Sultana (dried) Prune, Date Raisin (dried) Raspberry Red currant Loganberry Blackcurrant Youngberry Cherry Blueberry Orange Kiwi fruit Boysenberry Guava Blackberry Cranberry Apricot Strawberry Rockmelon Grape Plum Pineapple
Vegetables NEGLIGIBLE	LOW	MODERATE	HIGH	VERY HIGH
Potato (peeled) Lettuce Celery Cabbage Bamboo shoot Swede Dried beans Dried peas Red lentils Brown lentils	Green bean Red cabbage Brussels sprouts Mung bean sprouts Green pea Leek Shallot Chive Choko	Broccoli Sweet potato Parsnip Mushroom Carrot Beetroot Marrow Spinach Onion Cauliflower Turnip Asparagus Sweetcorn Pumpkin	Eggplant Watercress Cucumber Broad bean Alfalfa sprouts	Tomato products Gherkin Endive Champignon Radish Olive Capsicum Zucchini Chicory Hot pepper

Food Salicylate Content Table

NUTS				
NEGLIGIBLE	**LOW**	**MODERATE**	**HIGH**	**VERY HIGH**
Poppyseed	Cashews	Pistachio Pine-nut Macadamia Walnut, Brazil Coconut Peanut, Pecan Hazelnut Sunflower seeds Sesame seeds		Almond Water chestnut

Sweets				
NEGLIGIBLE	**LOW**	**MODERATE**	**HIGH**	**VERY HIGH**
Golden syrup Caramels	White sugar Maple syrup Cocoa Carob	Molasses		Liquorice Peppermints Honey

Food Salicylate Content Table

Herbs & Spices				
NEGLIGIBLE	**LOW**	**MODERATE**	**HIGH**	**VERY HIGH**
Vanilla Garlic Parsley Saffron Malt vinegar Soy sauce Tandori			Cinnamon Cardamom Black pepper Pimiento Ginger Allspice Clove Nutmeg Caraway White vinegar Bay Leaf White pepper	Cayenne Aniseed, Sage Mace, Curry Paprika, Thyme Dill, Turmeric Worcestershire sauce Vegemite Marmite Rosemary Mint, Oregano Garam masala Mixed herbs Cumin, Canella Tarragon Mustard Five spice

Alcohol				
LOW	**NEGLIGIBLE**	**MODERATE**	**HIGH**	**VERY HIGH**
	Gin Whiskey Vodka	Cider Beer Sherry Brandy		Liqueur Port Wine Rum

Anti-Inflammatory Diet

An unhealthy digestive tract always has excessive inflammation occurring in its tissues and this needs to be reduced by consuming an anti-inflammatory diet.

Foods to eat on an Anti-Inflammatory diet

Organic, free range and grass fed produce is much safer and healthier to consume, as it eliminates the use of toxic chemicals and unbalanced fertilizers as well as artificial hormones and antibiotics, which encourage inflammation in the gut. Try to find good reliable sources of this type of produce whenever possible or start your own vegetable and herb garden.

Vegetables

Raw and cooked. Make sure that you eat a rainbow of colors; cruciferous vegetables including Brussels sprouts, broccoli, cabbage, kale and cauliflower are especially high in antioxidants and detoxifying sulfur. Asparagus, beets, carrots, celery, cucumber, bok choy, green beans, leeks, mushrooms, mustard greens, okra, onions, garlic, parsley, peas, radishes, spinach, lettuce, sprouts, zucchini, watercress and sweet potato.

Fruits

Cherries and berries such as blueberries, blackberries, strawberries and raspberries are especially high in antioxidants and reduce inflammation. Papaya, apples, apricots, rockmelon, watermelon, pears, peaches, nectarines, plums, all citrus fruits, avocado and kiwi fruit.

Whole Grains

Choose gluten free such as buckwheat, quinoa, brown rice, black rice, wild rice, millet, amaranth, teff and buckwheat.

Protein

- Fresh cold water fish such as Alaskan salmon, oily fish such as sardines, trout, tuna, mackerel and halibut

- Organic free range chicken, duck and turkey

- Greek yogurt and white cheeses

- Free range eggs

- Lentils and legumes

Oils

Cold pressed extra virgin olive oil, coconut oil, flax seed oil, grape seed oil, hemp seed oil and avocado oil. Old oils can become rancid and oxidized, and so fresh is best. Store in a cool dark place.

Condiments

- Garlic, turmeric, cinnamon and ginger

- Green tea

- Organic apple cider vinegar

- Fresh herbs and spices

Seeds and Nuts

Almonds, sesame seeds, walnuts, Brazil nuts, macadamias, tahini paste, sunflower seeds, pumpkin seeds, freshly ground flax seeds, cashews, hemp seeds and chia seeds.

Foods to avoid on an Anti-Inflammatory Diet

- Refined or excess sugar

- If you have arthritis – you may have less pain if you avoid or minimize the nightshade vegetables such as eggplant, tomatoes, potatoes, capsicums (bell peppers), cayenne pepper and paprika

- Excess coffee and caffeinated drinks

- Sodas and diet sodas

- Alcohol

- Artificial food additives such as aspartame and MSG

- Refined grains such as white rice, white flour, white bread and pasta. Many people have less inflammation on a gluten free diet

- Trans-fats - these are found in commercially baked goods, "fast foods," deep fried foods, peanut butter with added vegetable oil, margarine and vegetable oils

- Meat from animals which have been fed processed stock feed (made with soy and corn etc.) and/or given artificial hormones and antibiotic drugs; meat produced this way can trigger inflammation. Grass fed beef and lamb can generally be considered safe and healthy. But some people find they have less inflammation when they go meat free. Avoid processed and preserved meats such as ham, bacon, salami etc. It is also best to avoid smoked meats and smoked fish because their fats have been oxidized.

Chapter 6

Recipes

Your Own Herb Garden

Your own herb garden can provide you with inexpensive fresh organic herbs, as well as great pleasure. Fresh herbs in particular taste so good and can even eliminate the need for added sauces, dressings and sweeteners. Herbs are very high in antioxidants and chlorophyll and improve the function of the liver. Many fresh green herbs have natural antibiotic and anti-cancer substances.

If fresh herbs are unavailable, dried herbs can be used, but fresh is always best.

Below are a few varieties of herbs that are easy to grow:

- Parsley - curly leaf and continental are both very easy to grow
- Basil - Vietnamese, Thai and bush basil are all delicious
- Chives - garlic and plain
- Garlic - standard or elephant (milder)
- Lemon-grass
- Rosemary
- Coriander - Vietnamese and standard
- Sage
- Oregano
- Dill and Fennel
- Mint

If you do not have enough ground area, most herbs grow well and look great in pots and hanging baskets. This is a good idea if you live in an apartment or unit and only have a porch or balcony.

Lemon-grass is a reed and grows well in a rockery or pot. Mature leaves can be used whole in cooking, then removed before serving or brewed in boiling water for tea - bulbs can be chopped finely or crushed with a tenderizer mallet and used for cooking.

Mint needs to be contained in a pot or basket as roots spread rapidly.

Good mint varieties are;

Spearmint - strong, rich sharp flavor and refreshing aroma.

Peppermint - stronger than spearmint with a hotter flavor

Apple mint - smaller softer leaf, milder more subtle flavor, definite apple smell- comes in plain green or green/cream variegated leaf.

Chocolate mint - is great for desserts and grows well in hanging baskets.

Parsley - all varieties of parsley do well in pots. They also look attractive in a rockery or cottage garden.

Sage - pineapple sage is a very attractive variety and bears bright green leaves with red sprays of small flowers. It is very tasty chopped into salads, stir fries, sweet and sour dishes, savory muffins, omelettes and quiches. It is best to use the young tender leaves.

Recipe Tips:

Ingredients such as flour, vegetables, fruits, nuts, lentils or liquids can be substituted, as long as they make up the same amounts as stated in the recipes. Herbs and seasonings should be used to individual taste and may be adjusted before serving. Many of these recipes are designed for more than one person. You can halve or double the ingredients if needed.

Special Note On Flour

All wholemeal SR (self raising) and plain flour can be substituted with other flours. For recipes that need SR flour use 1 teaspoon of baking powder plus the other flour.

For Gluten Free flour, a combination of buckwheat and soy flour, or rice, buckwheat and soy flour, works well. Using different flours will change the consistency of your muffin or pancake, however it will still be delicious. When plain flour is needed omit the baking powder.

Flaxseed

Much has been written about the benefits of flaxseed (linseed) in our diets and we now find it in many of our bread and cereal products. Since the introduction of LSA – a mixture of Linseed, Sunflower seeds and Almonds, many of us have added this mixture to our favorite recipes such as drinks, cereals, dips, cakes, biscuits, desserts, and in fact anything which can include a meal substance. LSA is an excellent source of healthy fatty acids, protein, minerals and vitamin E.

LSA

1 cup	*almonds*
2 cups	*sunflower seeds*
3 cups	*linseeds (flaxseeds)*

Use a coffee grinder or food processor to grind to a fine meal

Store in an airtight container in the refrigerator or freezer

Sprinkle over your usual cereal, on sandwiches, toast, or muffins with tahini, or nut paste and honey

If you only like fresh fruit for breakfast, chop up a banana, some melon, strawberries or any of your preferred fruit and sprinkle with LSA. This is the way to start your day with energy and avoid hunger until lunch time.

We can show you that just by using liver friendly foods and taking a little time to select recipes to suit your food tolerance, you will soon hear friends say, "Gee! You look well, you are lucky to be so healthy" Luck has nothing to do with it! Being healthy and looking good, is to do with you taking control of your own lifestyle and eating foods to help your liver perform its cleansing function.

A tip to get you through that between - meals - hunger - boredom- and cravings time - fill 2 x 1 litre carafes with drinking water, place one in the kitchen and one in your work space. If you find it difficult to drink lots of water, remember small quantities often, will soon get you in the habit of drinking more water. Try to drink water in between meals - this goes for tea and coffee as well.

Every night prepare a platter of bite size snacks. Place it center front top shelf of the refrigerator, so that it is easily seen when you are looking for nibbles. Keep the Platter, Simple, Varied and Fresh!

Carrot and celery sticks, snow peas, cauliflower florets and any other vegetable you like raw, a couple of pieces of fruit, grapes and small wedges of melon, some dried fruits and nuts. You cannot eat it all in one day and the variety will make you feel that you are not deprived of snacks. This will stop you from grazing on the wrong foods. Allow yourself no more than 3 - 4 of these snacks a day.

Healthy Beverages

Juices are so wonderful when they are freshly prepared and consumed straight away. However if you are time poor and would like to still have your daily dose of fresh juice, you could freeze larger quantities of the freshly made juice in glass jars and store it in your freezer to be consumed later. If you freeze your juice immediately after it has been extracted, most of its nutrients and antioxidants can still be retained for their healing benefits. You could also create frozen juice "icy poles" for a nice treat on a hot day as well. Kids can often be persuaded to get their daily dose of healing juice if it is given as a treat like an ice-block. It's worth a try! Here are some great juicy recipes to try out:

Juices Galore

Some simple combinations are;

- Carrot, fresh ginger and cucumber

- Carrot, celery, parsley, mint, tomato and apple

- Beetroot, apple, ginger and parsley

- Orange, lemon or lime (whole), carrot, fresh ginger and parsley

Juice for Inflammatory Bowel Disease

For disorders such as Ulcerative Colitis and Crohn's Disease

Basic Recipe:

1	Carrot
2	Celery sticks
2	Cabbage leaves or 2 kale leaves
5cm (2 inch)	Slice of beetroot
1	Apple or pear
½	Cucumber (skin on)
1 aloe vera leaf (spines removed)	

Optional extras to add to basic recipe:

2	Fresh Apricots or
½ cup	Chopped Fennel or
½	Papaya or
½ cup	Blackberries or
1 tsp	Glutamine powder

Tropical Smoothie to Heal the Bowel

1.5 cups	Coconut milk
1	Banana
1 tbsp	Slippery Elm Powder
1	Kiwi fruit or ½ cup blackberries or 6 strawberries or ½ paw-paw or 2 passion-fruit pulp. You may use less fruit if the diarrhea is bad.

If appetite is poor, you may add 1 tsp glutamine powder to this smoothie.

Place all ingredients into a blender and blend until smooth.

Juice to Assist Weak Digestion

1/3	Pineapple, skin on
1	Orange or ½ grapefruit
½	Cucumber
1	Apple, skin on
2 slices	Papaya

Trim the rough, dry pieces from the pineapple but retain as much green as you can. Thinly peel citrus leaving as much white pith as possible. Wash all ingredients and pass through the juicer. Drink twice a day, half an hour before meals.

Juice to fight Intestinal Parasites

2	Cabbage or Kale leaves
2	Spinach leaves
2	Apples, whole
1	Garlic clove or ½ red onion
1cm	Fresh ginger root
1cm	Horse radish root
2	Pomegranate (if in season) – seeds and flesh

Wash, trim and chop all ingredients and pass through the juicer.

Drink 300mls, three times daily. You may need to dilute the juice with water.

Juice for Irritable Bowel Syndrome

1	Apple, whole large
¼	Cabbage, medium sized
2	Celery sticks
1	Carrot
1cm	Fresh ginger root

Wash, trim and chop and process all ingredients through the juicer.

Drink 1 cup, twice daily

Smoothie for Irritable Bowel Syndrome

1 cup	*Rice, almond or coconut milk*
1	*Pear*
1 tsp	*Slippery Elm Powder*
1 tsp	*Glutamine powder*
2 tsp	*Ground flaxseed*
1 tsp	*Coconut oil*

Place all in a blender and blend until smooth.

Juice for Stomach Infections

(such as Helicobacter Pylori)

1	*Grapefruit, peeled but leave white pith on*
½ cup	*Cauliflower, chopped with stem and leaf*
1 cup	*Watercress*
2	*Cabbage leaves, green*
1	*Red radish with top leaves*
½ to 1	*Garlic clove (optional)*
1	*Pomegranate (when in season) – seeds and flesh*

Wash, chop and put all through the juicer.

Drink 1 cup, twice per day or more frequently if helpful. You may dilute with water or cold herbal tea.

Options:

1 medium carrot or 1 medium apple may be added for sweeter flavor.

Ginger is a natural remedy to settle the digestion and also addresses nausea.

Radish is a natural antibiotic and supports liver function.

Pomegranate reduces intestinal parasites such as worms, amoeba, giardia and helicobacter pylori.

Anti-Gas Juice

1cup	*Fennel, chopped*
1/3 cup	*Coriander leaves, chopped*
2	*Apples, whole with skin on*
2	*Celery sticks*

Wash, trim and chop and process all in the juicer. Drink 3 small glasses in between meals.

Anti-Hemorrhoid Juice

1 cup	*Watercress, chopped or 2 cabbage leaves or 2 turnip leaves*
1	*Large carrot*
2-3	*Spinach leaves and stems or 2 dandelion leaves*
1	*Garlic clove*
1	*Grapefruit or 1 orange with outside skin (pith) left on*

Wash, trim and chop, then process through juicer. Drink one glass twice daily.

Prune juice may also be drunk at breakfast to improve bowel habits. Soak dried prunes in water overnight, take out the stones and juice the fruit. You may also dilute juice with water, as increased fluid intake is vital to overcome hemorrhoids.

Smoothie for Peptic Ulcers

1	*Ripe Banana*
1	*Apple*
4	*Strawberries or 1 kiwi fruit*

1 tbsp	Slippery Elm powder (can use less if desired)
1 tsp	Glutamine powder
1cup	Coconut milk

Wash, trim and chop and process all in blender until smooth.

Constipation Smoothie

2	Spinach or Dandelion or Cabbage or Kale leaves
1	Green apple, whole, skin on
100 g	Dried prunes – stones removed
100 g	Figs, fresh if in season, otherwise dried
30g	Fresh Rhubarb
50 g	Fresh Cherries (stones removed) this is optional. Wash all fresh ingredients and chop to fit into blender. You will need a high powered blender (such as a Vitamix or Thermomix). Soak dried fruit in water overnight.

Options: Dilute with water to taste as the extra water will help the bowels. You can substitute stone fruits in season and also berries to make up the amounts.

Useful supplements include:

- FiberTone powder 2 tsp with breakfast.
- Ground flaxseed or LSA – 1 to 2 tbsp with breakfast
- Metamucil or Normacol

Mint Tea

2 tbsp	Chinese green tea
4 tbsp	Spearmint (or mint) chopped
900ml/32oz	Water
4 slices	Lemon or lime, thinly sliced

Honey or stevia or Nature Sweet Sugar Substitute to taste

Extra mint for garnish

Add tea and mint to a teapot.

Boil the water then pour into pot. Leave for 5 minutes.

Pour the tea through a strainer into warmed glasses. Add sweetener to taste and a slice of lemon.

Add sprig of mint for garnish.

Can be served hot or cold, poured over ice. Delicious!

Improves digestion and reduces risk of intestinal cancers.

Spiced Tea

6	*Cloves, whole*
2 strips	*Lemon rind*
1 stick	*Cinnamon bark*
2 tsp	*Tea (Formosan is nice)*
2 tbsp	*Fresh ginger grated*
5	*Lemon rings to serve*

Bring 5 cups of water, lemon rind, cloves, cinnamon and ginger to the boil.

Simmer for 10 minutes, then return to the boil. Pour the mixture into a teapot with the tea. Leave for 5 minutes. Strain and serve with lemon rind. A sweetener such as honey, stevia or Nature Sweet Sugar Substitute is optional

Recipe Legend

Gluten Free (GF)   *Free from wheat, oats, rye, barley, spelt*

Dairy Free (DF)   *Free from milk products from cows/goats*

Sugar Free (SF)   *Free from added sugars eg. table sugar, honey, agave, maple syrup etc.*

Nut Free (NF) Free from nuts and nut milks

Everyone is an individual when it comes to their gut

It must be noted that not all foods affect people in the same way. Extra care should be taken if you suffer from gastro-esophageal, intestinal or inflammatory bowel disease, (eg. Gastro-Esophageal Reflux Disease (GERD), Crohn's disease, irritable bowel syndrome (IBS), colitis and diverticular disease, to name but a few).

Keeping a daily diary of the foods you eat, and any symptoms you experience, is a practice I recommend. By keeping a record of your dietary intake, you can see which foods cause flare-ups or make you feel better.

Most recipes in this book will be tolerated quite well and will have an anti-inflammatory and healing effect on your condition. Conversely, some ingredients might intensify and irritate your symptoms. Since everyone is different, some ingredients in these recipes may have the potential to cause some symptoms and if so, OMIT them from the recipe. Some possible irritants may be fats and oils (even though they are healthy for you), chili or other spicy ingredients, grapefruit, oranges, tomatoes and dairy and gluten. The key here is to omit any ingredients you know may cause you increased symptoms.

Following is an example of a food diary which you may use to fill in and keep a record of your symptoms. This way it will become easier to see when any food item triggers off unpleasant symptoms. Once you are aware of these trigger foods, remove them from your diet.

Sample Food Diary

	SUN	MON	TUES	etc.
Food Diary for the Week of _____				
Breakfast	lemon water, poached eggs, salmon, spinach	lemon water, muesli, rice milk	lemon water, poached fruit, Greek yogurt	
Symptoms	nil	bloating, burping, flatulence	nil	
Snack	coffee, hummus, carrots	coffee, hummus, celery	raw juices	
Symptoms	nil	nil	nil	
Lunch	pumpkin soup, salad	mixed veg, egg, lentils, ryvita	mushroom salad, 2 slices bread	
Symptoms	nil	abdo pain, bloating	reflux	
Snack	mandarin	black tea, bean dip, celery	green tea, cake	
Symptoms	nil	fatigue	headaches, reflux	
Dinner	chicken kebabs, salad	tuna, potato salad, rice	lamb chops, steamed veg, salad	
Symptoms	nil	bloating, reflux	nil	
Snack	green tea, water, biscuit	strong black tea, water	water	
Symptoms	fatigue, coated tongue	excess stomach acid, burping	nil	

Breakfasts

Wild about Berries   (GF, SF, NF)

Serves 4 or more

1 cup	Raspberries, fresh
1 cup	Blueberries fresh
1 cup	Boysenberries, fresh
1 cup	Strawberries, fresh
1 cup	Mulberries or raspberries - frozen
300ml (10oz)	Greek dairy yogurt OR for a dairy free option try Coconut yogurt

Trim and wash berries. Slice strawberries and toss gently.

Place in individual serving comports.

Just before serving, whiz the yogurt and frozen berries together to make a whipped type of soft ice confection.

Serve and garnish with chopped mint.

Charles's Poached Eggs   (DF, SF)

Serves 1

2 large	Eggs, poached in simmering water
2 thick slices	Rye bread or sour dough bread toasted OR use gluten free bread, toasted
1	Tomato cut into halves and placed under griller
1 tbsp	Tahini paste
1 clove	Garlic, thinly sliced (optional)
1 tbsp	LSA (ground linseeds, sunflower seeds, almonds)
	Salt and ground black pepper to taste

Toast bread and spread thickly with tahini. The garlic goes next. Place poached eggs on toast and grilled tomatoes next to toast.

Sprinkle with LSA and garnish with parsley. Yum!

Poached Eggs with Salmon and Baby Spinach (GF, DF, SF, NF)

Serves 1

¼ cup	Vinegar
2	Organic or free range eggs
1 handful	Baby spinach
50g	Salmon
1 tbsp	Ground Flaxseeds

After filling a saucepan with water half way, bring the water to the boil.

Once boiling, reduce the heat to simmer.

Add ¼ cup of vinegar to the simmering water.

Create a whirlpool by stirring the water with a spoon.

Slowly add your eggs into the spinning water.

Poach your eggs for 1 minute if you prefer runny yolks or longer if a more solid egg is desired.

Place the baby spinach on a plate and top with the salmon.

Place the poached eggs on top of the salmon.

Sprinkle the dish with freshly ground flaxseeds.

Special note on flour

All wholemeal SR (self raising) and plain flour can be substituted with other flours. For recipes that need SR flour use 1 teaspoon of baking powder plus the other flour.

For Gluten Free flour, a combination of buckwheat and soy flour, or rice, buckwheat and soy flour, works well. Using different flours will change the consistency of your muffin or pancake, however it will still be delicious. When plain flour is needed omit the baking powder.

Muffins (Basic Recipe)

Makes approximately 12 muffins

1 large	*Egg*
1/2 cup	*Milk OR choose unsweetened almond or coconut milk*
2 tbsp	*Cold pressed olive oil or coconut oil*
1 tbsp	*Cabot Health Nature Sweet Natural Sugar Substitute or ½ tsp stevia*
1 cup	*Wholemeal SR flour OR for a gluten free alternative use *gluten free SR flour*
1 tbsp	*LSA (ground linseeds, sunflower seeds and almonds) or Hemp seeds*

Place egg, milk and oil in a bowl and whisk with fork.

Place flour in large bowl, make a well in middle and pour in liquid then sweetener

Mix gently. Place mixture in greased muffin tins.

Sprinkle tops lightly with cinnamon and sesame seeds.

Variations for muffins

Apricot   Add:

2 tbsp	*Plain yogurt to the liquid**
1/2 cup	*Dried apricots, chopped*
2 tbsp	*Shredded coconut*

Apple   Add:

1	*Apple, grated skin on*
1/2 cup	*Sultanas*
1 tsp	*Cinnamon - add to dry ingredients before mixing liquid*

Banana   Add:

| 1 | Banana, mashed |
| 1/2 cup | Walnuts – add to mixture |

Top with extra nuts or sunflower seeds.

Blueberry   Add:

| ½ | Punnet of fresh blueberries |

All variations are delicious served with a pile of berries on the side

Buckwheat Pancakes   (GF, SF)

Makes approximately 12 medium Gluten Free pancakes.

The pancakes can be either like pikelets or thin crepes

1 cup	Buckwheat flour
1	Egg
1/2 cup	Milk OR unsweetened rice or almond milk

Place flour into mixing bowl.

Add egg.

Pour in milk, half a cup first and stir.

Keep adding milk and whisking until the texture is heavy, but firm - like stiff cream.

Pour mixture into a hot fry-pan.

Cook until golden on either side.

Make a stack, cover with honey and lemon, or a mixture of berries, or poached eggs.

High Fiber Muesli   (DF, SF)

| 2 cups | Rolled Oats |
| 1 cup | LSA (ground linseeds, sunflower seeds and almonds) |

1 tbsp	Natural sultanas
2 tbsp	Chopped dried apricots
½ cup	Almonds, finely chopped
½ cup	Pepitas – ground or chopped
½ cup	Sunflower seeds – ground or chopped
½ cup	Hemp seeds (optional)

Mix all together and store in an airtight container. Stays fresher in the refrigerator.

1 serve = 2 to 4 tbsp of muesli with unsweetened milk (dairy, almond, rice or coconut milk)

Omelette Supreme   (GF, SF, NF)

Serves 2

3	Eggs
¼ cup	Milk
2-3	Spring onions, finely chopped
½ cup	Button mushrooms, thinly sliced
2 tbsp	Capsicum, finely chopped
2 tbsp	Sweet corn, fresh or canned and drained
1 tbsp	Parsley, chopped
1	Tomato, small, finely chopped
½ cup	Cheddar or Feta cheese, grated
2 tsp	Cold pressed olive oil

Salt and pepper to taste

Whisk eggs, parsley and milk together and set aside.

Heat the oil in a heavy based fry pan, add onion and capsicum and cook for 1 – 2 minutes.

Add tomato and corn and pour over the egg mixture, season to taste and sprinkle cheese on top.

Cook on medium heat until mixture is nearly set. Remove from the heat and place the pan under a griller to brown omelette and finish off the cooking.

Caution: Do not allow the handle of the pan to go under the griller.

Serve hot with a little grated carrot and beetroot and some alfalfa sprouts on the side.

Variation: Use ¼ cup of chopped sun-dried tomatoes instead of fresh tomatoes.

Low Carb Omelette (GF, DF, SF, NF)

Serves 1

2	*Fresh eggs*

Add a selection of fresh vegetables and meat that you enjoy such as chicken, avocado, salmon, tuna, broccoli (finely sliced), spinach, onion, chives, garlic, chili, coriander and other fresh herbs and sun-dried tomatoes (chopped). Black pepper and sea salt to taste.

Combine 2 eggs in a bowl and whisk, add all the other chopped ingredients and mix. Pour into a fry pan on low heat. Then flip the mixture in the pan and cook the topside or place under the grill to cook the top of the omelette.

Bubble and Squeak (GF, DF, SF, NF)

Serves 1

Use left-over mashed vegetables mixed together with 1 beaten egg and some finely chopped fresh herbs or dried herbs. Round them into patties and warm through on a fry-pan lightly brushed with olive oil. Serve with a non-sweetened relish, a piece of fresh fruit or a mixed raw vegetable juice.

Banana Crepes (GF, SF, NF)

Approx 12 or more crepes

Use a non-stick fry pan for this recipe, make the pancakes thin.

1 cup	*Buckwheat flour*
1	*Egg*
1/2 cup	*Milk OR use rice or coconut milk*
2 ripe	*Bananas*

Place flour into mixing bowl, add egg.

Pour in milk, half a cup at first, then stir. If required, add more.

Mash banana and add to mixture.

Add remaining milk and whisk until the texture is like heavy, but runny. Pour mixture into a hot fry-pan, cook until golden on either side. This is nice with fresh berries served on the side.

Poached Fruit (GF, DF, SF, NF)

Serves 2 - 3

6 small	*Pears*
2 strips	*Lemon peel, use a peeler*
1 cup	*Water*
1 tsp	*Cabot Health Nature Sweet Natural Sugar*

Substitute OR pinch stevia powder

Use a stainless steel or ceramic bowl.

Fill saucepan 1/4 full of water and place bowl on top.

Peel pears (any fruit will taste fantastic) and place in bowl.

Place lemon peel and water with pears.

The water in the saucepan will boil and the steam heats the bowl.

When the fruit is cooked, allow to cool.

Will store in the refrigerator.

Soups

Vegetable and Legume Soup (GF, DF, SF, NF)
Serves 8

This soup can be made with vegetable stock.

4 cups	Soup vegetables (swede, turnip, carrot and parsnip) grated
1 cup	Celery, chopped
2	Broccoli florets, chopped
1 cup	Soup Mix (mixed lentils and pulses often labeled Italian Soup Mix
1 cup	Brown lentils
½ cup	Kidney beans
1 cup	Onion, chopped
½ cup	Parsley, chopped
1 tsp	Pepper and sea salt to taste
1 tbsp	Cold pressed olive oil for browning onion

Soak all lentils, beans and soup mix in 3 cups of boiling water for 1 hour in a large saucepan.

Then add all other ingredients and enough soup stock to cover the ingredients.

Bring gently to the boil and simmer with lid on until everything is tender – about 1 hour, stirring occasionally and adding more stock if necessary. Season to taste.

This soup is rich and filling and substantial enough for a meal.

Suitable for freezing.

Dr Cabot Hint: If legumes cause intestinal gas take digestive enzymes with your meals. Sipping 1 tablespoon of apple cider vinegar in a small glass of water during meals can also improve digestion and reduce gas.

Tasty Chunky Tomato Lentil Soup (GF, DF, SF, NF)

Serves 6- 8

Suitable to freeze in meal size portions. This soup can be served chunky or if preferred smooth. For a smooth soup, purée with a hand held food processor or in a blender.

810g/29oz	Tomatoes, fresh and chopped
1 cup	Red lentils (soaked for 1 hour)
2 cups	Boiling water
1 cup	Celery, chopped
1 tbsp	Garlic, chopped
1 tbsp	Basil leaves, chopped fresh
1/2 cup	Parsley, chopped fresh
1 large	Onion, chopped
1 tbsp	Lemon juice
1/2 tsp	Sea salt
1/2 tsp	Pepper, freshly ground
1 tbsp	Tomato paste (or more)
1 tbsp	Cold pressed olive oil

Garlic and basil according to your personal taste

Pour the boiling water over the lentils and soak for 1 hour

Brown onion and garlic in oil in a pan

Add to other ingredients in a large pan

Simmer gently until all is tender, approx 1 hour. Add more water if necessary.

Season to taste

Serve sprinkled with chopped parsley.

Chicken and Vegetable Soup   (GF, DF, SF, NF)

Serves 6

4	*Chicken drumsticks, free range or organic is best*
2 cups	*Carrots, chopped*
½ cup	*Parsley, chopped*
1 cup	*Swede, grated*
1 cup	*Parsnip, chopped*
1 cup	*Celery, chopped*
400g can	*Whole corn, including liquid or use fresh corn sliced from cob*
1	*Large onion, chopped and browned in pan*

Place all ingredients in a large pan and barely cover with water.

Bring to the boil and simmer for 1 hour until tender.

Remove chicken bones and leave the meat in the soup.

Season with pepper and sea salt to taste.

Suitable to freeze in serving portions.

Pumpkin Soup   (GF, DF, SF, NF)

Serves 6

500g	*Pumpkin, peeled and cut into chunks*
125g	*Potato, peeled and cut into chunks*
1	*Large onion, thinly sliced*
1 cup	*Vegetable stock*
½ cup	*Fresh parsley, chopped*

Sea salt and cracked black pepper to taste

Place all ingredients in a large pan and barely cover with water.

Simmer until tender with the lid on for approximately 30 – 45 minutes.

Season to taste and place ingredients in a blender and puree.

Fish and Garlic Soup (GF, DF, SF, NF)

Serves 6 - 8

Any fish and/or your favorite shellfish can be used for this soup

2 sticks	Celery, sliced
2 large	Potatoes, chopped and peeled
1 whole	Chili, seeded, sliced (optional)
4 ½ cups	Stock, fish or vegetable
2 kg (4.4lbs)	Fish and shellfish prepared
2	Onions, chopped
10 cloves	Garlic, half thinly sliced, half crushed
6 med	Tomatoes, ripe, chopped
1 bunch	Dill, chopped
1 bunch	Parsley, chopped
1 bunch	Coriander
2	Lemons, juiced
3 tbsp	Cold pressed olive oil
	Salt and ground black pepper to taste

Brown onion, thinly sliced garlic and celery in oil for 2 minutes.

Add the crushed garlic and chili, cook for 1 minute.

Add potatoes, stir constantly till slightly golden.

Pour in stock and lemon juice.

Simmer until potatoes are tender.

Add fish, shell fish, tomatoes, herbs and seasoning.

Cook gently until seafood is tender.

Serve with a vegetable salad

Roast Tomato Soup

(GF, DF, SF, NF)

Serves 6

4 cups	Tomatoes, fresh, very ripe, chopped
1 large	Onion
4 cloves	Garlic
2 large	Potatoes, chopped
3 tbsp	Cold pressed olive oil
2 cups	Vegetable stock

Sea salt and cracked pepper to taste

Place all ingredients in baking pan

Bake in very hot oven until cooked

Put all the ingredients into a saucepan and purée

Heat slightly and serve

Tom Kha Gai Soup   **(GF, DF, NF)**

This healthy low carb soup is everyone's favorite Thai coconut chicken soup.

If you are currently experiencing gastritis or gut inflammation, please leave out the hot stuff - chili.

Serves 3

2 cans	Coconut milk
2 cups	Chicken stock
4	Red chillies, diced (optional*)
2.5cm	Galangal root, fresh, thinly sliced
2.5cm	Fresh ginger
2	Chicken breasts
1 can	Straw mushrooms

4 medium	Tomatoes (optional)
1 stalk	Lemon-grass, finely chopped (optional)
1 cup	Coriander (cilantro) fresh, chopped
10	Kaffir lime leaves, thinly sliced
3 tbsp	Lime juice
2 tbsp	Fish sauce
1 tbsp	Nature Sweet Sugar Substitute or brown sugar

Bring coconut milk and broth to a boil, add thinly sliced galangal, minced ginger, and chili to soup and simmer on medium for 10 minutes.

Add chicken slices and stir occasionally until chicken is tenderly cooked.

Add straw mushrooms (drained), and thinly sliced, deveined lime leaves. Cut a few cross-sections of lemon-grass and add to the soup. Cut tomatoes into 1 inch cubes and add to soup. Simmer for 10 more minutes.

Just before serving, turn off the heat, add coriander (cilantro), sweetener, lime juice and fish sauce and stir well.

Serve hot by itself or with rice.

Best to find an Asian grocer. You can substitute ginger root for the galangal root, and lemon peels for the lime leaves.

Dips, Spreads and Salad Dressings

Salmon or Tuna Dips   (GF, DF, SF, NF)

210g/8oz can	Pink salmon
2 tbsp	Tofu (fresh bean curd) crumbled
1 med	Onion, finely chopped
2 tbsp	Carrot grated
2 tbsp	Parsley, chopped
1 pinch	Chili powder (optional)

Mash fish and bones with a fork.

Mix in all other ingredients using enough of the fish juices to make a blended spread. You can blend finely in a blender if preferred.

Add a squeeze of lemon juice and salt and pepper to taste.

Piquant Fresh Herb Dip (GF, SF, NF)

1 cup	Natural plain or Greek yogurt
1 tbsp	Basil, chopped
1 tbsp	Parsley, chopped
1 tbsp	Chives, chopped
1 tbsp	Tomato paste
1 tsp	Dijon mustard
2 large	Garlic cloves, crushed (optional)
1/2 tsp	Cracked black pepper

Sea salt to taste

Combine all ingredients and mix well or blend finely in a blender if preferred.

Chill in refrigerator for a couple of hours to allow flavors to blend

Serve garnished with chopped parsley.

Hummus (GF, DF, SF, NF)

400g/14oz	Chickpeas, drained and rinsed (canned or cooked)
4 tbsp	Tahini
2 to 3 cloves	Garlic, crushed (more if desired)
2	Lemons juiced

Mix all together in a blender

Broad Bean Dip (GF, DF, SF, NF)

500g/18oz	Broad beans, frozen or fresh
1 tsp	Cumin powder
1 tsp	Cardamom powder
2 cloves	Garlic, crushed (more if desired)
1	Lemon juiced
1 whole	Chili, seeded and diced (optional)

Cook beans in water with cumin, cardamom and garlic. Drain beans and retain juice.

Add lemon juice and retrieve the garlic, place with the beans

Purée all together - add more juice if necessary

Serve warm with vegetable sticks or cold with crackers or on sandwiches.

Salad Dressing No 1 (GF, DF, SF, NF)

1 cup	Sesame oil, cold pressed
1 tbsp	Garlic, fresh, crushed
1/2 cup	Lemon juice
1/2 tsp	Cumin, dried

Put all ingredients into a jar, shake until well mixed. Store in refrigerator.

Salad Dressing No 2 (GF, DF, SF, NF)

1/2 cup	Apple cider vinegar (choose organic) or lemon juice
1/2 cup	Cold pressed olive oil
1 tbsp	Tamari
1 tsp	Mixed dried herbs or 1 tbsp fresh herbs, chopped

Put all ingredients into a jar, shake well until mixed, Store in refrigerator.

Salad Dressing No 3   **(GF, SF, NF)**

1/2 cup	*Plain or Greek yogurt*
1/2 cup	*Lemon or orange juice*
2 tbsp	*Mint, chopped*

Mix only as required.

Salad Dressing No 4   **(GF, DF, SF, NF)**

2	*Lemons, juiced*
3 tbsp	*Hummus, already prepared*
1 clove	*Garlic, crushed*
1 tbsp	*Cold pressed olive oil (optional)*

Mix all together in a jar

Salad Dressing No 5   **(GF, DF, SF, NF)**

1 tbsp	*Honey*
2 tsp	*Grainy mustard*
2 - 3 tbsp	*Cold pressed olive oil*
2	*Lemons, juiced*

Mix all together in a jar

Salads, Sides and Snacks

Sprouts, sprouts and more sprouts

There are some wonderful varieties of fresh sprouts - try a different one each week. Loosely separate the sprouts and gently toss together. Include one of the hotter varieties such as radish or mustard sprouts, and add just a little lemon juice to your taste. Prepare just the amount you need as this sprout salad is best eaten fresh.

NOTE: Remaining sprouts will store well in the fridge in the plastic containers in which they were packed and sold.

Salads are a mixture of raw fruits and vegetables. Salads do not have to have a dressing and many people prefer salads without dressing. If you are using ingredients that turn brown after they are cut, then you need to toss them in lemon juice, to stop this discoloration.

Salad garnishes

Vegetable waves

Using a vegetable peeler, carefully slice down the length of vegetables, such as carrots, Lebanese cucumbers, red and white radishes, zucchinis etc, so that you have long thin slices the length of your vegetable.

Vegetables such as carrots and radishes can be placed in really cold water for up to 30 minutes before use for extra crispness.

Vegetable curls

Cut sticks of vegetable about 6 cm long. Cut 2 or 3 slits with a sharp knife into one end of each piece. Stand in cold water in fridge for an hour and the end will curl - celery, carrot and radish are great for this.

Vegetable strings

Push grater length ways down vegetable to get long thin strings. Use crisp vegetables such as carrot, radish, beetroot and Japanese pumpkin.

Beetroot and Coriander Salad (GF, DF, SF)

Serves 3

1 bunch	Coriander (cilantro)
2 med	Beetroots, washed and peeled
4 tbsp	Lemon or lime juice
4 tbsp	LSA (linseeds, sunflower seeds and almonds) or hemp seeds

2 tbsp	Sunflower seeds, dry roasted and chopped
2	Carrots, washed and peeled

Wash and dice the coriander.

Wash and peel the beets and carrots.

Grate carrots and the beets. Be careful, as the red juice gets everywhere!

Put into a salad bowl. Add the LSA.

To roast the seeds -

Heat a small pan, add the sunflowers. Keep them moving. When they turn golden brown, take them off the heat. Pour the lemon juice over the salad.

Then toss on the hot sizzling sunflower seeds.

Gourmet Golden Pumpkins (GF, DF, SF, NF)

Serves 4 to 6

2 to 4	Golden nugget or butternut pumpkins
4	Garlic cloves, crushed
1 med	Onion, diced or 4 spring onions, chopped
1.5 cups	Brown rice, cooked
1/2 tsp	Coriander, ground
1/2 tsp	Cumin, ground
1 pinch	Nutmeg
2 tsp	Shoyu or tamari sauce

Cut small top off pumpkin and scoop out seeds, replace top.

Bake in moderate oven for 30 minutes, until tender.

Cool slightly and scrape out cooked pumpkin flesh from shell.

Take care not to damage the shell. Mix pumpkin and all other ingredients together - spoon back into the shell.

Drizzle a little sweet chili sauce on top of mixture (optional).

Hot, Crisp and Mellow Salad   (GF, SF)

Serves 4 - 6

15 small	Red radishes
1	Green apple, cored, quartered, thinly sliced
1 small	Mango, fresh, peeled and sliced
4 stalks	Celery, thinly sliced
1/2 cup	Walnuts, chopped

Dressing

1/2 cup	Plain or Greek yogurt
1 dstsp	Horseradish sauce
1 tbsp	Dill, freshly chopped
Salt and ground black pepper	
Fresh Dill for garnish	

Top and tail radishes, slice thinly.

Add to dressing with thinly sliced apple and celery and walnuts.

Peel, stone and cube mango, fold into mixture.

Garnish with dill.

Served chilled in a bowl.

Corn and Carrot Salad   (GF, DF, SF, NF)

Serves 4

2 med	Carrots, peeled
2	Corn cobs
3 tbsp	Sunflower seeds, dry roasted
4 small	Sweet potatoes, peeled

Dressing

2	Garlic cloves, crushed
2 tbsp	Lemon juice

| 1 tbsp | *Tamari* |
| 1 tbsp | *Tahini* |

Wash and peel all the vegetables.

Cut all vegetables into bite sized pieces.

Peel the corn and cut into thick rings.

Put all the vegetables into a steamer and cook until tender but still crisp.

Don't overcook them. Let cool and add the sunflower seeds.

For the dressing, mix all the ingredients together.

If it becomes too thick because of the tahini, add a small amount of water or lemon juice.

Big Green Salad   (GF, DF, SF)

Serves 4 - 6

Experiment with any green vegetables you enjoy.

1 bunch	*English spinach, washed and torn*
2 cups	*Snow peas, stringed*
2 cups	*Broccoli, florets*
2 bunches	*Asparagus*
1 cup	*Basil and parsley, chopped*
2 med	*Lebanese cucumbers, cut into thin strips*
1 med	*Capsicum green, seeded, sliced*
1 cup	*Green beans, cut in half*
4 tbsp	*LSA (linseeds, sunflower seeds and almonds)*

Wash all the vegetables.

Cut the tough bottoms off the asparagus and discard.

Put the broccoli, asparagus and beans into a steamer, cook until tender but still crisp.

Don't overcook them.

Tear up the lettuce and spinach and put into a large salad bowl.

Put the snow peas, capsicum and all the cooked vegetables into the bowl.

Toss in the herbs.

Serve with a dressing of your choice or with a lemon and cold pressed olive oil mix.

Nice cool salad   (GF, SF, NF)

To serve as a side dish with spicy foods

2	*Lebanese cucumbers*
1 large	*Carrot, washed and peeled*
2 tbsp	*Mint, chopped*
1/2 cup	*Plain or Greek yogurt, chilled*

Grate cucumbers and carrot.

Combine all ingredients.

Avocado Entrée or Light Meal   (GF, DF, SF, NF)

Serves 4

2 large	*Avocados*
125g/4-5oz tin	*Pink salmon*
1 dssp	*Tomato paste*
2	*Spring onions, tops finely chopped*
1	*Lemon juiced*
1 tbsp	*Soft tofu*
Tabasco sauce to taste	
Ground black pepper and sea salt to taste	

Cut avocados in half length ways. Scoop all flesh and mash into a bowl.

Mash drained fish and bones

Add mashed avocados with all other ingredients until evenly mixed.

Add a little of fish juice if necessary for smooth mix. Taste and add more seasoning if necessary.

Fill avocado shells with mixture.

Serve individually and garnish with slice of cucumber, tomato and alfalfa sprouts.

Savory Hash Browns (GF, DF, SF, NF)

Makes 6 - 12 hash browns

4 tbsp	Cold pressed olive oil
500g/18oz	Potatoes, lightly cooked and grated
1	Onion, finely chopped
1 tbsp	Mint, fresh chopped
1	Egg, beaten
Salt and black pepper to taste	

Mix all ingredients together, except oil.

Heat oil in a large pan, when hot add potato mixture.

Press flat and cook on moderate heat till golden brown, flip till golden.

Repeat till all the mixture is gone.

Serve anytime for, breakfast, snack, or as a side with meal. This is nice with grilled tomatoes and hot chili sauce (such as Cholula sauce)

Anytime Quick Asian Vegetables (DF, SF, NF)

Serves 4 or more

1/4	Cabbage, sliced
1 tbsp	Cold pressed oil (sesame seed, olive or coconut oil)
2 tsp	Ginger, fresh, grated
1/2 cup	Bamboo shoots
1/2 cup	Bean shoots

125g/4-5oz	Snow peas
100g/3-4oz	Field mushrooms
1	Red chili, chopped (optional)
1/2 cup	Water
1 tbsp	Tamari
2 cups	Chinese noodles (ready to eat)
	Cold pressed olive oil

Sauté ginger in oil in a large pan or wok.

Add cabbage and cook for 2 minutes tossing all the time.

Add all other vegetables and cook another 2 to 5 minutes.

Add to mixture with noodles, tossing all the time until all heated through.

Serve as a snack or side vegetable or cold as a salad.

Pumpkin Piquant Salad   (GF, DF, SF)

Serves 6

1 cup	Blue pumpkin, grated or in thin strips
4	Spring onions, thinly sliced diagonally
1/3 cup	Raisins
1/2 cup	Walnuts or pecan pieces
1 tbsp	Fennel - fresh, thinly sliced
1 med	Orange, peeled and cut into chunks
1 tbsp	Mint, chopped
1 tbsp	Lemon juice
1 clove	Garlic, crushed

Mix all together, cover and stand in refrigerator for about an hour.

Serve with dressing no 1 (see page 172)

Mixed Vegetable, Egg and Lentil salad

(GF, DF, SF, NF)

Serves 6 to 8

1 large	*Carrot, cut into thin strips*
200g/7oz	*Broccoli florets*
300g/11oz	*Cauliflower florets*
2 sticks	*Celery, cut into thin slices*
6 baby	*Potatoes, steamed*
400g/14oz	*Lentils, drained and halved*
1 small	*Red capsicum*
2 tbsp	*Garlic chives fresh, chopped*
2 tbsp	*Oregano, fresh, chopped*
2 tbsp	*Mint, fresh chopped*
6	*Eggs, hard boiled and chopped*
10	*Snow peas, trimmed*
3/4 cup	*No 1 dressing – (see page 172)*

Steam carrot, broccoli and cauliflower until cooked but still crisp.

Cool and mix all other ingredients together except the dressing.

Cover in bowl and refrigerate overnight.

Fold dressing through before serving.

Serve with a bowl of delicious roast vegetables.

Sweet Savory Salad **(GF, DF, SF, NF)**

Serves 4 or more

1 cup	*Watermelon, balled or diced*
1 cup	*Rock melon (cantaloupe), balled or diced*
1 cup	*Honey-dew melon, balled or diced*
1 cup	*Mint, chopped or if you prefer parsley*

¼ cup	Pumpkin seeds, chopped
¼ cup	Hemp seeds (optional)
1/4 cup	Sesame seeds, toasted
1/4 cup	Lemon or orange juice

Mix all ingredients gently together.

Let stand in refrigerator, in an airtight container for 1/2 hour to allow flavors to blend.

Serve individually in small lettuce cups on a large platter.

Sweet Corn Salad   (GF, DF, SF, NF)

Serves 4 - 6

2 cups	Corn slices from the cob, fresh, young and juicy
1 large	Red apple
2 tbsp	Mint, fresh, chopped
4	Spring onions, thinly sliced
1	Naval orange, peeled and cubed
1 large	Lemon, juiced ground black pepper to taste

Take leaves and fibers from corn cobs.

Use a sharp knife remove corn niblets carefully, keep the niblets whole.

Core and dice apple leaving skin, toss immediately into lemon juice.

Mix all ingredients together and serve.

Cool, Refreshing Cucumber Salad (GF, DF, SF, NF)

Serves 4 or more

4 small	Cucumbers, Lebanese or small continental
1	Red onion, finely chopped
1 tbsp	Mint, chopped fresh
1 small	Green capsicum, thinly sliced
1 large	Tomato sliced finely

1/2 cup	Apple cider vinegar – choose organic
1/3 cup	Cold pressed olive oil
Sea salt and ground black pepper to taste	

Wash cucumbers, score skins with a fork, rinse then slice thinly.
Mix all ingredients and toss together.

The purpose of life is to discover your gifts.
The meaning of life is to give your gifts away with love.

Greens 'n' Things   (GF, DF, SF, NF)

Serves 6 - 8

1 cup	Broccoli florets
1 cup	Celery, diced
1 cup	Green capsicum, diced
1 cup	Green beans, chopped
6	Spring onions, tops and all chopped
1 cup	Snow peas, trimmed
1 cup	Parsley, fresh chopped
1 cup	Cucumber, Lebanese or small continental
A few red cherry tomatoes to garnish	
Sea salt and black pepper	

Blanch broccoli in boiling water for 1 minute, drain, rinse.
Score cucumber skin with a fork, rinse under cold water and dice.
Toss all ingredients together with no 1 dressing – see page 172.

Tabouli with Silver Beet   (DF, SF, NF)

4 or more

1 cup	*Burghal (cracked wheat)*
1 cup	*Mint, fresh chopped*
1 cup	*Parsley, fresh chopped*
1 large	*Onion, finely chopped*
4 small	*Young silver beet or Spinach leaves*
1/2 cup	*Lemon juice, fresh squeezed*
1/2 cup	*Cold pressed olive oil*
1 cup	*Red cherry tomatoes (more if desired)*

Ground black pepper to taste.

Soak burghal in 2 cups warm water for about 3/4 hour.

Strain and pat dry on some paper toweling.

Soak silver beet leaves until they are crisp, trim stalks roughly chop.

Mix burghal, mint, parsley, onion and silver beet together.

Combine juice and oil and toss through salad.

Add pepper to taste then add cherry tomatoes.

Mushroom Plus Salad   (GF, DF, SF)

Serves 4 - 6

250g/9oz	*Button and field mushrooms, thinly sliced*
1/2 cup	*Cashew nuts, chopped*
1 small	*Red capsicum, seeded and thinly sliced*
1 cup	*Mung bean sprouts*
2 tbsp	*Garlic chives, chopped*
1 tbsp	*Tamari*
3 tbsp	*Cold pressed olive oil*

Sea salt ground black pepper to taste.

Mix all ingredients together until combined.

Gently toss in enough no 3 dressing until all ingredients are lightly coated.

Tomato Salad   (GF, DF, SF, NF)

Serves 4 or more

Great to eat as a snack with bread or serve with any mains hot or cold.

6	*Roma ripe tomatoes (long Italian variety)*
3 tbsp	*Basil leaves, chopped, fresh*
1	*Onion, small, chopped*
2 - 3 cloves	*Garlic, crushed*
1 tsp	*Oregano, ground or 1 tbsp fresh chopped*
1/2 cup	*Lemon or lime juice, fresh squeezed*
3 tbsp	*Cold pressed olive oil*
Fresh sea salt and ground black pepper to taste	

Cut tomatoes.

Sprinkle with oregano, stand for 15 minutes.

Add all other ingredients.

This combination gives tomatoes an exceptional flavor.

Boiled Egg Salad & Avocado Dressing

(GF, DF, SF, NF)

Serves 4 or more

6	*Eggs, hard boiled, cut into quarters*
	Paprika to garnish

Dressing

1/2 cup	*Orange juice, fresh squeezed*
1/4 cup	*Lemon juice, fresh*

1 large	Avocado, peeled and stoned
1	Garlic clove, crushed
1 tbsp	Fresh mint, chopped

Mix dressing ingredients in a blender until smooth.

Pour over eggs and sprinkle with paprika.

Simply Carrots   (GF, DF, SF, NF)

Serves 2

Great on sandwiches, pocket pita bread and tacos. Will keep in a sealed container in the refrigerator for1 or 2 days.

1 cup	Carrots, grated or julienne sliced
1/2 cup	Green beans, chopped or peas (cooked)
3 tbsp	Water cress, chopped
2 tbsp	Orange juice, fresh
	Grind some black pepper to your taste

Mix all ingredients together and serve

This salad is not only good for your liver, it will also improve your eyesight.

Greens with Almonds and Zesty Lemon Dressing   (GF, DF, SF)

2 bunches	Broccolini
2 bunches	Asparagus
150g	Sugar Snap peas
¼ cup	Almonds

Dressing

2 tsp	Olive Oil, cold pressed
1tsp	Lemon rind, grated
1 tbsp	Fresh Lemon juice

Place olive oil, lemon rind and lemon juice in a glass jar with a lid and shake to combine.

Lightly roast or dry fry the almonds over medium heat. Steam the broccolini, asparagus and sugar snap peas for 1 minute. Place the steamed vegetables on a serving platter. Top with the roasted almonds and then drizzle the lemon dressing over the veggies.

Coleslaw Supreme (GF, SF, NF)

Serves 4 - 6

2 cups	Cabbage, finely shredded (Savoy or Chinese)
1 cup	Red cabbage, finely shredded
1 med	Onion, thinly sliced in half rings
1 cup	Whole corn, sliced off cob
1 cup	Carrot, grated or fine julienne strips
1/2 cup	Parsley, roughly chopped
1	Lemon, juiced

Sea salt and black pepper to taste

Dressing

1/2 cup	Natural plain yogurt or Mayonnaise
1/4 cup	Orange juice, fresh
1/4 cup	Apple cider vinegar or lemon juice
1 tsp	Chili or Hot English mustard or other mustard you enjoy (optional)

Ground black pepper to taste

Blend all ingredients in dressing together. Toss dressing through coleslaw salad

Special Potato Salad   (GF)

Serves 4 or more

750g /27oz	New baby potatoes
1	Red onion, thinly sliced in half rings
3 cloves	Garlic, crushed
4	Hard boiled eggs, chopped
3 tbsp	Mint or coriander, fresh, chopped
2 tbsp	Almonds, roasted, sliced

Dressing

1/2 cup	Natural plain yogurt
1/2 cup	Light malt vinegar or lemon juice
1 tsp	Honey, warmed for easy mixing

(Alternatively use Cabot Health Nature Sweet Natural Sugar Substitute or Stevia instead for a sugar free dressing)

1 tsp	Dijon mustard

Sea salt and ground black pepper to taste

Mix dressing ingredients together until all combined

Wash potatoes, leave skin on and cut in half, cook until just tender

Gently mix all ingredients together then pour dressing all over

Beaut Beetroot Salad   (GF, DF, SF)

Serves 4 or more

1 cup	Beetroot, washed and trimmed
1 med	Onion
1 large	Orange, peeled of all pith
1/2 cup	Pine nuts or walnuts
1	Garlic clove, crushed

Beetroot is best if coarsely grated or in very thin julienne strips.

Slice onion into thin 1/2 rings.

Slice orange into thin 1/2 slices.

Toss all ingredients into bowl.

Add dressing no 2 (see page 172) just before serving.

Great with BBQ's, chicken or grilled fish

Spicy Tomato Bake (DF, SF, NF)

Serves 4 or more

2 large	*Onions, cut into very thin rings*
820g/30oz	*Tomatoes, canned or fresh, chopped*
1 tbsp	*Basil, fresh, chopped*
1 tbsp	*Cold pressed olive oil*
2 cups	*Breadcrumbs (or Gluten free bread crumbs or Rice crumbs*), fresh*
1 tsp	*Mixed dried herbs*
3	*Garlic cloves, crushed*

Salt and ground black pepper to taste

Separate onion rings and place in casserole dish.

Mix basil with tomatoes, then place on top of onions

Rub oil into breadcrumbs and mixed herbs.

Sprinkle breadcrumb mix on top of tomatoes.

Bake casserole in a moderate oven for about 40 minutes until onion is tender and topping is golden brown

Mashed Potato with a Difference (GF, SF, NF)

Serves 4 or more

Ideal to serve with fish in place of chipped potatoes.

500g/18oz	*Potatoes, peeled, chopped and cooked in unsalted water until tender*

1 tbsp	*Natural plain yogurt*
2	*Spring onions, finely chopped*
2 tsp	*Horseradish mixed in a little plain yogurt*

Sea salt and ground pepper to taste.

Mash drained potato, yogurt and enough milk to make a smooth mixture.

Add onions, horseradish, salt and pepper.

This can also be placed on top of a casserole. Rough the top of the potato with a fork and place under a griller until golden brown.

Stuffed Baked Capsicums (GF, DF, SF, NF)

Serves 4

2 large	*Red capsicums, cut into halves and deseeded*
1 cup	*Rice, cooked*
1 large	*Tomato, ripe, chopped*
4	*Garlic cloves, crushed*
1/2 tsp	*Ground coriander*
1/4 tsp	*Chili powder (optional)*
1 med	*Onion, finely chopped*
1 tbsp	*Tamari*

Place capsicum halves in an oven-proof dish

Mix all other ingredients together and spoon into capsicum halves

Cover dish with foil

Bake in a moderate oven for 1/2 hour or until vegetables are tender

Vegetarian Mains

Stir Fry Beans with Lemon and Cashews

(GF, DF, SF)

Serves 2 - 4

This is a delicious dish when beans are in season and preferably when they are organic or home grown!

2 tbsp	Cold pressed olive oil
1 handful	Green beans, trimmed
1 handful	Yellow beans, trimmed
1 handful	Snow peas, trimmed
2	Garlic cloves, finely sliced
3/4 cup	Unsalted cashews
1 large	Lemon, juiced
2 tbsp	Tamari
2 tbsp	Mint (laksa) leaves
1 tbsp	Ginger, fresh grated
1 tbsp	Lemon-grass, finely chopped
2 cups	Rice, cooked

Heat 2 tbsp olive oil in wok.

Add garlic and cashews and stir fry for 1 minute.

Add all beans and continue cooking for another two minutes or until crisp and tender.

Add ginger, lemon-grass, tamari and laksa mint and fry for another minute or two, until all ingredients are blended.

Serve immediately on a bed of freshly steamed rice that has been cooked in vegetable stock, or water and a clove of garlic

Tomato and Fennel Risotto   (GF, DF, SF, NF)

Serves 2 - 4

Risotto is a meal in itself, for those craving a creamy textured meal. It is worth adding to your repertoire, although it may feel time consuming, when mastered you'll never look back!

6	*Roma tomatoes, slice length ways, place on oven tray*
440g/16oz	*Tomatoes, canned and mashed*
3 cups	*Vegetable stock*
2 large	*Brown onions, coarsely chopped*
2	*Garlic cloves, crushed*
3	*Baby fennel, sliced finely (around 1cm / 1/2 inch)*
2 cups	*Italian Arborio rice*
1/2 tsp	*Rosemary, dried*
	Olive oil for stir frying and roasting

Drizzle olive oil over tomatoes, sprinkle with rosemary, cracked pepper and some sea salt.

Place in a moderate oven and roast until golden brown.

In a heavy based saucepan, add two tablespoons of oil, and heat.

When hot, add onions and garlic and stir fry for 2 minutes.

Add the Arborio rice and stir fry until clear, add the fennel and stir.

Add tinned tomatoes and stir into mixture and simmer.

Put the stock into a jug and slowly add it to the mixture while stirring. Continue adding stock and stir until all the liquid is absorbed and the rice is soft and the risotto is creamy in texture (if you need more liquid use some extra vegetable stock).

Season with pepper and sea salt

Serve on a plate with the roasted Roma tomatoes piled on top.

Susan's Summer Pasta Salad (DF, SF, NF)

Serves 4

1/2 cup	Cold pressed olive oil
500g /18oz	Tomatoes, firm and ripe, finely chopped
2 small	Onions, finely chopped
10	Green olives, pitted and chopped
6	Black olives, pitted and chopped
2	Garlic cloves, crushed
1/3 cup	Parsley, fresh, finely chopped
1 tbsp	Capers
1/4 tsp	Oregano, fresh, finely chopped
2 tbsp	Sesame seeds, toasted
1 packet	Wholemeal pasta or Gluten free pasta such as buckwheat or rice pasta

Cook the pasta.

Combine all ingredients into a bowl.

Mix well, allow mixture to stand overnight, in the refrigerator.

Sprinkle with toasted sesame seeds and serve cold mixture over warm pasta.

Basic Tomato Pasta Sauce (GF, DF, SF, NF)

Serves 4

2 cups	Tomatoes, fresh or canned, chopped
1	Onion, thinly sliced
2	Garlic cloves, minced
1 tbsp	Tomato paste
1 cup	Vegetable stock or water
1 cup	Parsley, chopped

Black pepper and sea salt to taste

Heat fry pan, add tomato paste and stir for 1 - 2 minutes

Add oil, onion, garlic and cook for approx 5 minutes Add tomatoes, and water or stock, cook for 10 minutes Just before serving, add the parsley, stir in for 30 seconds

A basic sauce, experiment with other flavors, ie. chili, bay leaves etc

Vegetable Stew   (DF, SF, NF)

Serves 4

1 bunch	*Asparagus, trimmed and cut into lengths*
8 small	*Zucchini, ends trimmed*
12	*Baby carrots, trimmed and peeled*
8	*Onions, peeled*
1 cup	*Peas, fresh from the pod*
6 baby	*Turnips, peeled and topped*
1	*Shallot, peeled and finely chopped*
700ml/24oz	*Vegetable stock*
2 med	*Tomatoes*
2 tbsp	*Cold pressed olive oil*
15	*Basil leaves*

Salt and black pepper to taste

Blanch the asparagus, zucchini, carrots, peas, turnips and onions separately in salted water. Don't overcook them, they must be quite crisp.

Drain and run under cold water.

In a large pan, sauté the shallots in 2 tbsp of oil.

Add stock and bring to the boil.

Simmer to reduce the quantity of water by at least half.

Add diced tomatoes.

Simmer for 3 minutes

Add the remaining vegetables and heat for a further 4 minutes.

Season with salt and pepper.

Sprinkle with the basil and serve in shallow bowls.

Serve with toasted Turkish bread (or gluten free bread) and a big green salad.

Chunky Roast Vegetables (GF, DF, SF, NF)

Serves 4

This dish is also great cold!

2 large	Capsicums (Peppers) yellow and red, seeded, cut into thick strips
4 small quarters	Eggplants, trimmed, cut length ways into
6 small	Potatoes, cut into halves
3 med	Onions, peeled and cut into quarters
2 bunches	Asparagus, hard ends cut off
10 cloves	Garlic, whole, peeled
6	Thyme sprigs
4	Rosemary sprigs
3 tbsp	Olive oil
Salt and ground black pepper	

Preheat the oven to its highest setting.

Put all the vegetables into two trays.

Toss in the garlic and herbs, over the two trays.

Season with salt and pepper.

Drizzle oil (olive oil or coconut oil) over the vegetables, lightly.

Bake for approx 20 - 30 minutes in a moderate oven.

Serve alone, or with a big salad or grilled fish.

Stroganoff without Meat (GF, SF, NF)

Serves 4

440g/16oz	Lima beans, canned, drained, rinsed,
1 tbsp	Raw garlic, crushed
440g/16oz	Tomatoes, canned
1 med	Onion, chopped
2 med	Zucchini, grated
1 cup	Broccoli, chopped
1 med	Capsicum, seeded, cut into thin strips
2 tbsp	Tomato paste
1/2 cup	Vegetable stock
400g/14oz	Button or field mushrooms, washed
1 cup	Plain yogurt
1	Bay leaf

Sea salt and cracked pepper to taste

Combine all ingredients except mushrooms and yogurt.

Place in a covered casserole dish

Bake in a moderate oven for 45 minutes.

Add mushrooms and cook further 15 minutes.

Before serving, stir in yogurt.

Serve with a big green salad

Spicy Pasta (DF, SF, NF)

Serves 4

250g/9oz	Dry wholemeal pasta OR gluten free spiral pasta
1 large	Carrot, cut into thin strips
1 stick	Celery, cut into thin slices

1	Red capsicum, cut into thin strips
1/2 cup	Broccoli, chopped
1/2	Green beans, chopped
4 small	Chillies, whole stems on
1/4 cup	No 2 dressing see- page 172
1 tsp	Curry paste of your choice
2 tsp	Turmeric powder

Add pasta to boiling water and boil uncovered until pasta is just tender, drain.

Steam vegetables until crispy but tender, drain.

Mix dressing and spices together and gently toss through pasta and vegetables.

Serve with a big green salad and crusty bread

Broad Beans   (GF, DF, SF, NF)

Serves 4

If you have never enjoyed broad beans before, give this a try because these beans are delicious and have many health benefits

500g /18oz	Broad beans - fresh or frozen
440g/16oz	Tomatoes, canned or fresh and chopped
3	Garlic cloves, crushed (optional)
2 tbsp	Basil, fresh chopped (mint if you do not like basil)
1 large	Onion, chopped
	Ground black pepper and sea salt to taste

Cook beans until tender then drain.

Brown onion and garlic in pan with a little cold pressed olive oil. Add beans and tomato to pan and add basil and simmer for 5 minutes. Season to taste

Tangy Tasty Lunch - Mexican Style

(GF, SF, NF)

Serves 4 - 6

450g/16oz	Red kidney beans, canned, drained or cooked
1 large	Onion, chopped
3 large	Garlic cloves, chopped
1 tbsp	Cold pressed olive oil
1 tbsp	Tomato paste (more if desired)
1 tsp	Oregano, fresh
1 tbsp	Parsley, fresh chopped
1 tbsp	Basil, fresh chopped
1 pinch	Chili powder and paprika (optional)
A little water	
Sea salt and cracked pepper to taste	

Brown onion and garlic in oil in large pan.

Add all other ingredients plus enough water to bind together.

Don't make it too moist, warm through.

Serve with rice, chopped tomatoes, sliced lettuce, alfalfa sprouts.

Add some chilled Greek yogurt.

Basic Vegetable Stock

(GF, DF, SF, NF)

5 cups	Water
5	Black peppercorns
1	Onion, skin on and cut in half
2	Carrot, whole
2	Tomato, washed and halved
2	Bay leaves
2 stalks	Celery

| 1 tsp | Sea salt |
| 2 tbsp | Cold pressed olive oil |

In a hot heavy saucepan, add oil.

When hot, add all ingredients except water

Keep ingredients moving so they don't stick and burn, for 5 minutes.

Add water, bring to the boil, then simmer for an hour.

Strain.

Use immediately or cool, then refrigerate.

Nori Rolls   (GF, DF, SF)

Makes approx 10 rolls

You will need a sushi mat for this recipe, which you can get from some supermarkets or an Asian grocery store. Try using different ingredients like prawns, tofu, tuna and salmon. Great for lunches, entrées and snacks.

5 sheets	Nori seaweed
1 med	Avocado
1 bunch	Garlic chives
2	Lebanese cucumbers
3 tbsp	LSA (linseeds, sunflower seeds and almonds – ground)
2 tbsp	Sesame seeds, dry roasted
1 tube	Wasabi (horseradish paste)
1 pkt	Pickled ginger (optional)
4 tbsp	Tamari
5 cups	Brown or basmati rice, cooked

While the rice is still warm stir through the LSA and sesame seeds.

Let the rice sit while you prepare the other ingredients.

Peel the avocado and slice into strips.

Wash and separate the garlic chives.

Cut the cucumber into long thin strips.

Put the nori sheet on the sushi mat and cover the nori with a thin layer of rice.

Leave about 2cm (3/4 inch) clear at the top and bottom of the nori. Fill to the sides.

Spread a thin strip of wasabi along the center of the rice.

At the end closest to you, place 3 strips of garlic chives.

Put a strip of cucumber next then a strip of avocado.

Roll the mat up, away from you, creating a compact roll. Be careful not to roll the mat into the nori roll.

You can cut the long rolls into bite size pieces or just in half. Use a wet knife to do so.

Serve with pickled ginger, a dipping sauce of wasabi stirred into the tamari and a big green salad

Tempeh Salad (GF, DF, SF, NF)

Serves 2

390g/14oz	Tempeh
1 cup	Bean sprouts
1	Green chili
3	Spring onions
2 tsp	Ginger root, grated
2	Garlic cloves, crushed
1 tbsp	Apple cider vinegar or lemon juice
1 tbsp	Tamari
1/2 tsp	Mustard (optional)
6 tbsp	Water
4 tbsp	Cold pressed olive oil

Ground black pepper and salt to taste

Cut the tempeh into thin strips. Wash the bean sprouts.

*Heat the oil and stir fry the tempeh until golden brown.
Set the tempeh aside*

In the same pan, stir fry the spring onions, chillies, ginger and garlic for about 1 minute.

Add the water and bring to the boil.

Turn the heat down and simmer for 2 minutes.

Add the tempeh, stir and add the bean sprouts.

Simmer for a further 2 minutes.

Serve hot or cold on a bed of rice with a big salad

Poultry

Stir Fry Chicken with Lime Leaves (GF, DF, SF, NF)

Serves 4

A tasty stir fry with the clean fresh taste of kaffir lime leaves

2 tbsp	Sesame oil or coconut oil
6	Shallots, finely chopped
1 tbsp	Ginger, freshly grated
8	Lime leaves (try kaffir lime leaves), finely shredded
4	Free range chicken fillets, sliced into thin strips
3 tbsp	Tamari
1 tbsp	Red miso
2 bunches	Bok choy (Asian, green leafy vegetable)
4 tbsp	Basil, torn
2 cups	Rice, cooked

In a wok, heat sesame oil and add shallots, ginger, lime leaves and chicken.

Add the tamari, miso and bok choy and stir through.

Keep the wok moving over heat, cook until the chicken is tender.

Stir through basil and serve on a bed of steamed rice.

(Try cooking the rice with coconut milk instead of water for an authentic Asian flavor!)

Serve with a green salad

Cooking Hint for Stir-fry

The secret to a good stir fry is to heat the wok first, add the oil or stock (if you would rather avoid the oil). Add the ingredients immediately to the oil, so that the oil does not get burnt. Keep the heat high and the food moving in the wok.

Summer Chicken Kebabs (GF, DF, SF, NF)

Serves 4

Something for the BBQ or under the grill on balmy summer nights

4	*Chicken breast fillets, cut into bite sized pieces*
24	*Button mushrooms*
1 large	*Onion, cut into bite size pieces*

8 Stainless steel or wooden skewers from the supermarket

Marinade

1/3 cup	*Cold pressed olive oil*
2	*Chillies, fresh finely sliced (optional)*
2 tbsp	*Coriander, fresh chopped*
1 tsp	*Ground turmeric*
1 tsp	*Ground cumin*
2 tbsp	*Tamari*
1 tbsp	*Lime or lemon juice*

Combine all marinade ingredients into a large bowl and stir well.

Add chicken pieces to marinade, cover and refrigerate for 2 hours.

When ready to cook, take a skewer and thread chicken, onion pieces and mushrooms alternately, until all 8 skewers are prepared

Barbecue, or grill, turning occasionally for 8 mins or until chicken is tender

Serve with your favorite summer salad

Alternatively you could replace the chicken with fish, lamb and/or tofu!

Chicken Omelette **(GF, DF, SF, NF)**

Serves 2

4 large	Eggs, free range
1 med	Zucchini, grated
1 cup	Chicken fillets, cut into thin strips
2 tbsp	Fish sauce
2 tsp	Sambal (chillies in vinegar), or fresh chili (optional)
1 cup	Chicken stock
1	Spring onion tops, chopped.

Peanut or cold pressed olive oil for frying

Use a fry-pan or wok.

Put half oil, heat and quickly cook the chicken.

Remove the chicken from the pan.

Crack the eggs and put into a mixing bowl.

Put the zucchini, chicken and fish sauce into the bowl.

Whisk or beat the ingredients.

In the wok, place 1 tbsp oil, heat and swirl around.

Place half the ingredients and swirl around, flip over when brown.

Repeat for the other side.

Do exactly the same for the other omelette.

Heat the chicken stock.

Add 1 teaspoon of sambal (optional but delicious).

In 2 small bowls pour the chicken stock and sprinkle with spring onions

Serve with a large side salad

Grilled Chicken and Fig Salad (GF, DF, SF, NF)

Serves 2-4

A dish to enjoy for lunch or dinner

2 large	*Chicken breasts*
1	*Eggplant sliced in 1cm (1/2 inch) rounds*
8	*Radicchio leaves (a bitter yet tasty lettuce style plant, with purple blush to the leaves)*
6	*Fresh figs, halved*

Cold pressed olive oil for cooking

Dressing

1 med	*Lemon, freshly squeezed juice*
½ cup	*Marjoram leaves*
1	*Garlic clove, crushed (optional)*

Dash of Tamari

In a jar, squeeze the juice of one medium lemon. Add the marjoram leaves and a dash of tamari, sea salt and pepper to taste.

Put a lid on the jar and shake until well combined and set aside.

Baste the chicken fillets and eggplant in olive oil and grill until chicken is tender and eggplant is golden brown (the chicken may need to go under the grill first).

Wash and pat dry radicchio leaves.

Arrange two leaves on each of 4 plates.

When chicken and eggplant is cooked, slice chicken into long thickish strips.

Pile chicken and eggplant onto leaves and top with fresh figs.

Shake dressing and pour onto salad

For best results serve while still warm.

Poached Chicken Breasts with Spring Vegetables (GF, DF, SF, NF)

Serves 4

300ml/10oz	*Chicken stock*
2	*Garlic cloves, crushed*
4	*Chicken breasts*
1 tbsp	*Basil pesto (already prepared)*
1 bunch	*Watercress, washed and set aside*
1 tbsp	*Chives chopped*
100 g/4oz	*Baby carrots, washed*
100 g/4oz	*Broad beans, shelled*
6	*Baby zucchini, topped tailed, sliced length way*

Salt and pepper to taste

Put chicken stock, watercress, pesto, some salt and pepper into a food processor.

Blend until smooth.

In a large saucepan place the zucchini, baby carrots and broad beans.

Sprinkle with garlic and chives.

Lay the chicken on top of the vegetables.

Pour the sauce over the top and cover.

Simmer for 30 to 40 mins or until chicken is tender.

Chicken and Vegetable Stir Fry   (DF, SF, NF)

Serves 4 - 6

The dried mushrooms are necessary for the flavor. Quantities of vegetables can be added or taken out as desired

1 tbsp	Cold pressed olive oil
2 tbsp	Tamari
1200 ml/40oz	Chicken stock
6 to 8	Shiitake mushrooms, soaked in warm water, 30 mins or field/button mushrooms
3	Chicken fillets, sliced finely
8 fresh	Asparagus spears, chopped into 2.5cm (1inch) pieces
12	Green beans, chopped into 2.5cm (1 inch) pieces
14	Sugar snap peas, washed
1 handful	Bean and/or snow pea sprouts
125g/4-5oz	Noodles, yellow Asian noodles, boiled for 2 minutes

Warm the stock in a large saucepan while you cook the stir fry.

Just before you begin cooking, put the cooked noodles into the warming stock to heat before serving.

Heat the oil in a wok or deep fry-pan.

Add asparagus and beans and stir fry for 2 mins.

Add chicken and fry for another 2 mins.

Drain the mushrooms, add to stir fry along with peas.

Stir for another two mins.

Stir through tamari and bean sprouts and turn off heat

Place equal portions stock and noodles into large soup bowls.

Put spoonfuls of stir fry into the bowls.

Warm Chicken Salad (GF, DF, SF, NF)

Serves 3 - 4

Positively lip smacking!

4 tbsp	Cold pressed olive oil
2	Garlic cloves, crushed
500g/18oz	Cherry tomatoes, washed
4	Lebanese cucumbers, cut thinly length ways
200g/7oz	Artichokes, tinned, drained and quartered
100g/3-4oz	Caper berries, drained (small)
3	Chicken breast fillets, poached and sliced
2 tbsp	Basil leaves, chopped
3 tbsp	Organic apple cider vinegar or lemon juice
1	Bay leaf
4 tbsp	Chicken stock or water

To Poach Chicken

In a non-stick fry-pan, add 4 tablespoons of chicken stock or water along with the bay leaf, and bring to the boil.

Place the chicken breasts into the pan and reduce the temperature down to a gentle simmer, until cooked.

Combine tomatoes, cucumber, chicken, caper berries, artichokes and herbs into a large bowl.

Combine olive oil, cider vinegar or lemon juice, and garlic and pour over salad.

Gently mix salad and set aside.

Serve on large platter or individual plates.

Season with salt and pepper to taste

Singapore Noodles (DF, SF, NF)

Serves 4 - 6

3 tbsp	Cold pressed olive oil
3	Garlic cloves, crushed
2	Red chillies, finely chopped (optional)
3	Spring onions, finely chopped
250ml/8oz	Fish stock
250g/9oz	Chicken, cooked thinly sliced
300g/11oz	Small prawns
2 tsp	Salted soy bean paste, mixed with 1 tbsp water, or 3 tsp soy sauce without adding extra water
2 cups	White Chinese cabbage (bok choy), sliced finely cross ways
500g/18oz	Hokkien mee noodles
250g/9oz	Bean sprouts
1 handful	Baby spinach leaves
2 tbsp	Tamari

Heat oil in wok or large pan and stir fry garlic until golden.

Remove garlic from pan with slotted spoon and set aside for garnish.

Stir fry the chillies in the oil then add prawns and soybean paste.

Stir fry for 2 minutes then add cabbage and spring onions.

Add fish stock, noodles, bean sprouts and spinach leaves.

Continue to cook and simmer for 2 minutes, turning slowly Stir through tamari and put into individual bowls.

Garnish with garlic and cucumber for a rewarding flavor combination!

Thai Green Chicken Curry (GF, DF, SF, NF)

Serves 4

350g/12-13oz	Chicken, chopped into pieces
1 tbsp	Thai green curry paste (you might like more)

1 tbsp	Cold pressed olive oil or coconut oil
1 cup	Green peas (fresh)
1 cup	Green beans, tipped and left whole
1 cup	Coconut cream
1/2 cup	Coriander
1 tbsp	Lemon, chopped very finely
2 whole	Red chillies (optional)
2 cups	Rice, cooked

Heat oil in a pan on medium-low heat.

Add curry paste and heat for one minute.

Add half the coconut milk and cook until oil appears on the top.

Add chicken pieces and cook for around 10 minutes or until done.

Add the remaining coconut milk, green peas, beans and lemons.

Simmer until tender.

Garnish with sprigs of coriander.

Serve with boiled rice and fresh garden salad

Apricot Fat-Free Chicken (GF, DF, SF)

Serves 4

4 large	Chicken breast fillets, trimmed of all fat
4 tbsp	Dried apricots, chopped
2 tbsp	Hazelnuts, chopped
1 tsp	Dried oregano (if fresh, triple the amount and dice)
2	Garlic cloves, chopped
	Sea salt and freshly ground black pepper to taste

Mix apricots, nuts and oregano.

Cut the chicken fillets to open out as flat as possible.

Lay one fillet out and sprinkle 1/4 of filling over the flesh, repeat for the other 3 fillets.

Sprinkle top fillet with ground black pepper and a little oregano.

Tie fillets into a parcel shape with string and place into oven bag.

Add 2 tablespoons of apricot nectar or water to oven bag.

Bake in oven as directed - about 1 hour or until tender.

After cooking, snip bag and retain juices, make juices up to 1 cup with water, and use as a tasty sauce

Slice your chicken parcel carefully with a sharp knife

Basic Chicken Stock (GF, DF, SF, NF)

500g/18oz	*Chicken, wings, bones, legs (choose free range)*
5 cups	*Water*
5	*Black peppercorns*
1	*Onion, skin on and cut in half*
1	*Carrot, whole*
2	*Bay leaves*
2 stalks	*Celery*
1 tsp	*Sea salt*
2 tbsp	*Cold pressed olive oil*

In a hot heavy saucepan, add oil.

When hot, add all ingredients except bay leaves and water.

Keep ingredients moving so they don't stick and burn, for about 5 minutes.

Add water and bay leaves, bring to the boil, then simmer for an hour.

Strain and let cool and scrape off the fat.

Refrigerate or reheat to use.

Seafood

Scallops with Grape Fruit Juice (GF, DF, SF)

Serves 4

2	Garlic cloves, crushed
1 cup	Grapefruit, juiced
4	Spring onions, finely sliced
1 tsp	Cold pressed walnut oil (or olive oil)
48	Fresh scallops on ½ shell

Combine garlic, grapefruit juice, onion and oil.

Place scallops in shells in a single layer on an oven tray.

Spoon some of the mixture over scallops.

Add freshly ground pepper and grill for 5 minutes.

Toss in a bowl with remaining juice and devour. Serve with a tossed salad and steamed potatoes.

Grilled Korma Curry and Spiced Snapper

(GF, DF, SF)

Serves 4

2 whole	Baby snapper, cleaned and gutted
1/3 cup	Korma Curry Paste
1/2 cup	Slivered almonds
1/2 cup	Coriander leaves, chopped finely
1	Lime, cut into wedges for garnish
1 tbsp	Cold pressed olive oil

Slice each snapper on both sides 3-4 times diagonally

Preheat grill or barbecue

In a small bowl combine together the Korma curry paste, slivered *almonds and coriander and baste over fish*

Grill snapper on both sides until center is cooked

Brush citrus pieces with oil and lightly grill- serve with snapper

Serve with rice and salad.

Tuna and Potato Salad   (GF, DF, SF, NF)

Serves 2 or more

1/4 cup	Cold pressed olive oil
2 tbsp	Tamari (wheat free soy sauce)
1	Red salad onion, peeled and sliced finely
225g/8oz	Tuna
1/2	Iceberg lettuce, washed and torn up
1	Garlic clove, crushed
1	Lemon juiced
1	Lebanese cucumber, sliced length ways
1 punnet	Cherry tomatoes, washed
8 small	Tomatoes, chopped
4	Eggs, hard boiled and quartered
8 small	New potatoes, steamed, left to cool, then quartered

Combine oil, tamari, lemon juice and some salt and set aside.

Put remaining ingredients into a large serving bowl and mix gently.

Pour dressing over salad and set aside for 5 mins before serving.

Tuna and Rice Hotpot   (GF, DF, SF, NF)

Serves 4

4	Tuna steaks
1.5 cups	Basmati rice
1/2 tsp	Sea salt

3 tbsp	Cold pressed olive oil
1/2 tsp	Chili powder (optional)
2 tbsp	Lemon juice
2	Onions finely chopped
450g/16oz	Button mushrooms sliced
2 tbsp	Fresh ginger, grated
2 large	Tomatoes, skinned and chopped
450g/16oz	Spinach washed/shredded
2 - 4 large	Red chillies seeded (optional)
2 cups	Fish stock or water

Ground black pepper and sea salt to taste

Soak the rice in cold water for 2 hours (makes it soft). Rub the tuna with salt, chili powder and lemon juice Put the steaks on a plate in the fridge.

To make salsa -

Stir fry onions in the oil until soft. Add mushrooms, cook for 1 minute. Add chillies, ginger, tomatoes and seasoning, cook for another 5 minutes. Set aside in a cool place until needed.

Drain the rice.

In a large pot with a tight fitting lid put the stock or water and rice, bring to the boil. Turn the heat down, simmer for 10 minutes.

Place half the spinach on top of the rice, then half of the tomato salsa, then the tuna steaks.

Repeat the spinach and finally the tomato salsa on top.

Cover the top tightly and cook for another 15-20 minutes.

Remove from the heat and let it sit for 5 minutes on a damp tea towel.

Serve with a big green salad.

Tuna or Salmon Salad (GF, DF, SF, NF)

Serves 4

250g/8oz	Tuna or red salmon in brine
1 handful	Black olives, pitted
8 large	Lettuce leaves, washed and torn up
2	Spring onions, finely sliced
2	Eggs, hard boiled and halved
3	Tomatoes, ripe and diced

Dressing

1 tbsp	Cold pressed olive oil
1 tbsp	Tamari
1	Lemon, juiced

In a large bowl combine all ingredients, except the eggs

Shake dressing and pour over salad

Add eggs and season to taste. Simple as that!

Marinated Fish with Grapefruit, Noodles and Asparagus (GF, DF, SF)

Serves 4 - 6

2	Grapefruit, peeled and segmented
1	Grapefruit, juiced
1 tbsp	Organic apple cider vinegar or lemon juice
1	Garlic clove, crushed
1/2 cup	Sesame oil, cold pressed
1/4 cup	Walnut oil or cold pressed olive oil
4	Spring onions, finely sliced (chill in cold water to curl onion, drain, set aside)

1kg/36oz	Tuna or salmon steaks, slice across the grain, as fine as possible (try partially freezing the steaks to make slicing easier)
1 tsp	Cold pressed olive oil
1 bunch	Asparagus spears, trimmed and halved (blanched in boiling water and set aside)
250g/9oz	Rice noodles

Combine grapefruit juice, cider vinegar, garlic, walnut, sesame oil, and half the spring onions into a bowl.

Place the fish steaks in a shallow ceramic dish, pour over half the marinade (refrigerate for 2 hours or longer, turn the steaks at least once).

Cook noodles in a large saucepan of boiling water for 5 mins. Drain and rinse under cold water.

Toss noodles in olive oil.

In a fry pan, quickly sear the fish steaks on both sides

Pile the noodles onto a plate and place fish steaks on top

Place the grapefruit, asparagus and remaining green onions onto the steaks

Spoon on remaining marinade

Serve on a large platter as part of a banquet or with a big vegetable salad

Red Curry Fish Cakes (GF, DF, SF, NF)

Serves 12

1tbsp	Cold pressed olive oil
500g	White flesh fish fillets, already precooked
2tsp	Lime juice
1tbsp	Coriander, ground
½ bunch	Coriander, fresh

2tbsp	Sesame seeds
2tbsp	Coconut cream
1tbsp	Red curry paste
3	Spring onions
1	Egg yolk

Cut the white fish into chunks or small pieces.

Combine all other ingredients with the fish and stir well to ensure everything is mixed well.

Take approximately two dessert spoons of the mixture and shape into a patty.

Place onto a plate ready for cooking.

Heat the olive oil in a pan and fry or BBQ the fish cakes until browned.

Turn the cakes over and cook on the other side until cooked through.

Serve with fresh salad and/or a favorite dipping sauce.

Fresh Fish with Ginger and Spring Onions

(GF, DF, SF, NF)

Serves 4

Tuna, Atlantic salmon or salmon trout are the preferred choices for this refreshing meal.

Try wrapping the fish in fresh banana leaves instead of foil. Available at Asian green grocers and in some supermarkets.

4 pieces	Fish of your choice, fresh
4 tsp	Cold pressed olive oil
3	Spring onions, sliced cross ways
1 piece	Ginger, freshly grated
4 pieces	Foil or banana leaves for wrapping fish

Thinly sliced lemon wedges for garnish

Preheat oven to 180 deg C or 350 deg F.

Place a piece of fish onto the foil or leaf.

Spoon over 1 teaspoon of oil, some ginger, spring onions and a lemon wedge.

Loosely cover with foil or wrap in banana leaves.

Repeat the process 3 more times for other pieces of fish.

Place all parcels in an oven proof dish.

Bake for 15 to 20 minutes.

When ready season with salt and pepper to taste.

Serve with a fresh cucumber salad.

Marinated Calamari (GF, DF, SF, NF)

Serves 4

This dish is best made the day before you need it.

500g/18oz	*Calamari (small tubes are more tender)*
1/3 cup	*Cold pressed olive oil*
2	*Garlic cloves, finely chopped*
1/3 cup	*Lemon juice*
2 tbsp	*Parsley, chopped*

Wash squid under cold running water and pat dry. Slice squid into 1cm (1/2 inch) rings.

Bring a large saucepan of water to the boil and drop in the squid.

Reduce the heat and simmer for 5 minutes, drain and set aside.

In a bowl, combine oil, lemon juice and squid. Cover and refrigerate overnight.

When ready to serve, add the garlic and parsley to the marinade.

Mix well and let stand for two hours, season to taste.

Serve in the marinade at the table with a big green salad!

Basic Fish Stock   (GF, DF, SF, NF)

2 kg/4.4lbs	Fish including bones and heads (white fish), rinsed
2 tbsp	Cold pressed olive oil
1	Carrot
2 stalks	Celery
10	Black peppercorns
3 strips	Lemon peel
5 cups	Water
1/2 bunch	Parsley with stems

Heat heavy saucepan, add oil, fish, carrot, celery, parsley, peppercorns and lemon peel and add water.

Bring to a simmer, cover and turn down the heat.

Skim off the foam.

Cook for approx 45 minutes, then strain through muslin or sieve.

Use straight away or store in the refrigerator.

Grilled Sardines with Lemon   (GF, DF, SF, NF)

Serves 4

1kg/36oz	Sardines, fresh (filleted)

Marinade

6 tbsp	Cold pressed olive oil
2	Garlic cloves, finely chopped
1/2 cup	Lemon juice
4 tbsp	Coriander, chopped
	Salt and black pepper to taste

Mix up the marinade.

Brush the fish with oil and pour half the marinade on each side.

Brush with marinade each turn,

Serve with the remaining marinade poured over the top and a vegetable salad or a big green salad and Turkish or gluten free bread served on the side.

Hint to Prepare Fish

To descale the fish, use the back of a knife and scrape the scales off.

Cut off fins with scissors. Slit along the stomach, remove and discard intestines.

Wash well, pat dry and place in ceramic or plastic dish

Thai Seafood Casserole   (GF, DF, NF)

Serves 6

The fish markets or your local market would be the best place for your fresh ingredients to make this dish.

2 kg/70oz	*Seafood, mixed fresh (include white fleshed fish, green prawns and crab)*
12	*Black pepper corns*
1	*Kaffir lime leaf*
5	*Garlic cloves, finely chopped*
5	*Coriander roots, washed and trimmed*
1 cup	*Coconut cream*
4	*Spring onions, finely sliced*
4 fresh	*Green chillies, finely sliced (optional)*
3	*Red chillies, finely sliced (optional)*
6 stalks	*Lemon grass, finely sliced*
3 cups	*Coconut milk*
4 tbsp	*Fish sauce (anchovies, water and salt)*
1 tbsp	*Maple syrup or 1 tsp Cabot Health Nature Sweet Natural Sugar Substitute*

Wash and cut up seafood into bite sized pieces.

Use a mortar and pestle to crush coriander, garlic and peppercorns into a paste.

Use a vegetable peeler to remove a thin strip of the lime skin to use for later

Squeeze lime juice into a cup.

Put coconut cream into heavy based saucepan, slowly bring to boil.

Add the paste and simmer for 5 mins.

Add spring onions, green chillies, lemon-grass, lime rind, coconut milk and bring back to the boil.

Add seafood, stir in fish sauce, lime juice, nature sweet or syrup and simmer gently. Remove seafood from pan when cooked, transfer to warm serving dish. Season to taste and adjust the balance between sweet, salty and sour.

Spoon enough mixture over seafood to just cover.

Serve sprinkled with red chillies. (optional)

Fresh Fish with Beetroot (GF, DF, SF, NF)

Serves 4

1 kg/36oz	Tomatoes, quartered
1	Garlic clove, crushed
1 cup	Basil leaves, roughly chopped
2 tbsp	Dill, fresh, finely sliced
6	Baby beets
1	Red (luscious) capsicum
4	Tuna or salmon steaks (approximately 150 g/5-6oz each)
1	Lemon, juiced
	Cold pressed olive oil for roasting

Grease a shallow baking dish with oil and put in the tomatoes.

Baste tomatoes with a little oil and salt.

Cook for 40 minutes in 180C/350F oven.

Remove from oven and sprinkle with dill and basil then set aside to allow flavors to meld.

Slice capsicum length ways into 4 pieces, then char under a grill until skin blisters and turns black.

Then place capsicum in a plastic bag and allow to cool; then you can peel off the skin.

Put crushed garlic and some oil onto capsicum.

Cook beets in salty boiling water until tender; when cooked. Cut into quarters, length ways.

Drizzle beets with oil and lemon juice and set aside.

Sear fish steaks in hot fry pan, about one minute each side.

Divide ingredients into 4 servings.

Pile the beetroots onto plate and top with capsicum and tuna steaks.

Add tomatoes

Serve garnished with basil and a garden salad!

Squid with Savory Rice   (GF, DF, SF, NF)

Serves 4

4 med	Squid tubes, cleaned
2 cups	Rice, cooked
2	Onions, chopped
3	Garlic cloves, crushed
1 tbsp	Cold pressed olive oil
1/2 cup	Chives, chopped
1 large	Lemon, juiced
1 pinch	Chili powder (optional)

1 med	Red capsicum, chopped
440g/16oz	Tomatoes, tinned, chopped
1/2 cup	Basil, fresh, chopped

Little extra olive oil

Salt and ground black pepper to taste

Brown onion and garlic in 1 tablespoon oil.

Add 1/2 can of tomatoes, rice and all other ingredients, except chopped basil.

Stuff the squid tubes with the rice mixture and lay flat in casserole dish. Retain excess rice mixture.

Drizzle extra oil over squid then top with remaining tomato.

Cover dish and cook in a medium oven until tender, about 1 hour. Test with a skewer.

Heat and divide remaining rice mixture on to 4 serving plates.

Serve sprinkled with basil, fresh tomato wedges, pitted black olives and sliced cucumber.

Individual Fish Cutlets   (GF, DF, SF, NF)

Serves 4

4	White fish cutlets (snapper or similar)
1 small	Red capsicum
1 small	Green capsicum
1 med	Zucchini
1 stick	Celery
1 tsp	Cumin, ground
1 tsp	Ginger, freshly grated
1 tsp	Dill leaves, chopped
2 tbsp	Lemon juice
1 tbsp	Cold pressed olive oil

Salt and ground black pepper to taste

Banana leaves or foil for wrapping

Cut vegetables into thin strips.

Heat oil in pan.

Stir in cumin, capsicum, zucchini, celery and dill.

Stir and cook for further 2 minutes.

Place each fish cutlet onto a large sheet of foil, or a leaf. Sprinkle with lemon juice.

Divide vegetable mixture over fish.

Wrap fish in the foil or banana leaves.

Place in medium oven for about 25 minutes or until fish is cooked.

Remove foil and serve with small boiled potatoes and a green salad.

Fish Steaks with Tangy Topping (GF, DF, SF, NF)

Serves 4

Tangy topping can be served either hot or cold.

4	White fish steaks
2	Tomatoes, seeded and chopped
4	Spring onions, chopped
1 tbsp	Basil, chopped
2 tbsp	Parsley, chopped
1 tbsp	Lemon juice
1 tbsp	Cold pressed olive oil
	Salt and ground black pepper to taste

Cook fish under grill, 4 to 5 minutes each side. Keep warm until serving

Combine all other ingredients in bowl to make tomato mixture

Serve fish topped with tomato mixture, on a bed of rice or noodles and a big green salad

Anchovy Sauce (GF, DF, SF, NF)

Serves 4

A fairly thick sauce to serve with polenta or pasta

1 small tin	Anchovy flat fillets in oil
2	Garlic cloves, crushed
1 tbsp	Tomato paste
6 tbsp desired	Basil and parsley freshly chopped, more if
1	Onion, chopped
1.5 cups	Vegetable stock
400g/14oz	Tomatoes, chopped
2 tbsp	Cold pressed olive oil

Sea salt and ground black pepper to taste

Brown onion and garlic in oil, add tomato paste cook for 3 minutes.

Add anchovies and their oil, tomatoes, stock and herbs.

Cook until the anchovies have disappeared, approximately 20 minutes.

Grilled Atlantic Salmon with Mash (GF, SF, NF)

Serves 4

3	Red capsicums cored, cut into quarters
1 tbsp	Balsamic vinegar or lemon juice
2 tbsp	Cold pressed olive oil
220g /8oz	Atlantic salmon, fillets (4 fillets)
4	Tomatoes cut in half

freshly ground black pepper

Mashed potatoes

600g/21oz	Potatoes, peeled, quartered
2 tbsp	Cold pressed olive oil

1/3 cup	Milk or (for dairy free try Almond or soy milk)
2 tbsp	Horseradish

Preheat oven to 180C/350F.

Place capsicums and tomatoes in baking dish.

Cover with oil and balsamic vinegar.

Add pepper and bake for 30 minutes.

Cook salmon under preheated grill for approx 4-5 minutes each side.

Cook potatoes until soft and drain.

In a pot, mash potatoes with milk and oil and stir in the horseradish. Spoon mashed potatoes and roasted capsicums and tomatoes (with juices) onto warmed plates.

Top with salmon

Serve with a garden salad.

Chili and Lime Snapper   (GF, DF, NF)

Serves 4

2 tbsp	Cold pressed olive oil
2 tbsp	Ginger, grated
1 tbsp	Fish sauce
½ - 1 tsp	Cabot Health Nature Sweet Natural Sugar Substitute or Stevia
2 tbsp	Lime juice
2 tbsp	Sweet chili sauce (optional)
2	Garlic cloves, crushed
2 bunches	Baby bok choy, separate leaves and wash
4	Snapper fillets washed
1 cup	Coriander leaves washed,
Steamed jasmine or basmati rice	

Combine chili sauce, lime juice, oil, sweetener, ginger, garlic and fish sauce.

Add all but 2 tablespoons of mixture to a wok and bring to the boil.

Add bok choy, cover and cook.

Stir until leaves are bright green and stalks feel tender (around 2 minutes). Remove from heat and keep warm.

Brush the fish fillets with the left over lime juice mixture.

Grill for 2 to 3 minutes on each side.

Serve fish sprinkled with coriander leaves on a bed of rice.

Place bok choy on the side of the rice.

Pasta Verdi   (DF, SF)

Serves 2 - 4

This pasta dish is made with fresh green herbs and gives you a mineral and vitamin boost to boot!

You need a food processor for putting ingredients in directly

10 sprigs	*Chives fresh*
2 handfuls	*Flat leaf parsley*
1bunch	*Fresh basil*
10	*Rocket leaves*
1 handful	*Dill fresh*
4	*Anchovies*
1 tbsp	*Capers*
2	*Garlic cloves, crushed*
1/2 cup	*Pine nuts*
1/2 cup	*Cold pressed olive oil*
1 packet	*Pasta of your choice OR (gluten free pasta)*

Olive oil for blending

Prepare a large saucepan with enough water to boil your pasta then place on the heat.

Put 1/2 cup olive oil into food processor (you can use less).

Add remaining ingredients, blend until greens are puréed.

If you need more oil add it now. There should be enough oil to create a sauce.

The pasta sauce is now done you simply have to wait until the pasta is cooked (normally 10 minutes).

Serve pasta in a big bowl and stir sauce through it for a flavorsome treat!

Meat

Some people may be surprised to find recipes including red meat in a book that advocates healthy eating for the liver and bowels. Many people today believe that red meat is unhealthy because it contains saturated fat and is a very concentrated source of animal protein. Others believe that red meat is higher in bacteria than plant food and some avoid it for philosophical reasons. However if you enjoy red meat, provided it is very fresh and is thoroughly cooked, red meat does not present any greater risk of bowel infection than eating chicken or seafood. Grass fed animals raised in countries with clean soils is an excellent source of low carbohydrate protein, omega 3 fatty acids, healthy cholesterol and iron.

I have included some healthy red meat dishes that can be prepared in a liver friendly manner, and served with liver cleansing foods to support the liver to process animal meats. We encourage you to use only fresh lean cuts of meat and preferably meat that is grass fed. Always cook the meat very well so that the middle of the meat is cooked thoroughly, as this will kill bacteria. Do not eat meats that are preserved or smoked and make sure that you buy only the freshest meat available.

Curried Beef and Beans   (GF, DF, SF, NF)

Serves 4

500g/18oz	Lean beef (preferably rump), cubed
440g/16oz	tomatoes, canned
440g/16oz	Borlotti beans, canned, drained
1 large	Onion, chopped
2 tsp	Red curry paste(more if desired)
1 tbsp	Garlic clove, crushed
1 dstsp	Ginger, freshly grated
1 tsp	Chili, fresh, diced, no seeds (optional)
1 tsp	Turmeric
1/2 large	Lemon, juiced
2 tbsp	Mint, freshly chopped
1 tsp	Garam masala
2 tbsp	Cold pressed olive oil

Brown beef cubes in hot oil until tender, set aside.

Sauté onion, garlic and ginger.

Add all other ingredients except beans and simmer for 3 minutes.

Stir in beef and beans

Cover pan and simmer for 3 to 5 minutes.

Serve with cooked brown rice, steamed greens and carrots.

Taste to season before serving.

Quick Beef and Mushroom Casserole
(GF, DF, SF, NF)

Serves 4 - 6

750g/27oz	Lean beef strips (rump is ideal)
1 large	Onion, cut into rings

1 tbsp	Cold pressed olive oil
1 med	Red capsicum, seeded and chopped
150g/5oz	Field mushrooms
2 cups	Water
2 tbsp	Tomato paste
2 tsp	Oregano, fresh and chopped

Heat oil in large pan, brown beef, onion and capsicum, stir often.

Add all other ingredients, cover pan, Simmer for about 40 to 45 minutes.

Serve with rice, steamed carrots, snow peas and a big green salad.

Piquant Lamb Steaks (GF, NF, SF)

Serves 4

4	Lamb fillets or leg steaks
2 tbsp	Plain full fat yogurt
2 tsp	Horseradish sauce
1 tsp	Hot chili sauce (optional*)
1 tsp	Capers, drained and chopped
1	Onion, chopped
½ - 1 tsp	Cabot Health Nature Sweet Natural Sugar Substitute or Stevia
1 tbsp	Garlic chives, chopped

Cold pressed olive oil for browning meat.

Heat oil in pan and cook lamb for 5 minutes on each side.

Mix all other ingredients together, spread on each side of lamb.

Cook for a further 5 minutes on each side or until tender.

Serve with steamed baby potatoes sprinkled with chopped garlic chives, steamed zucchini and snow peas

Spicy Beef with Pulses (GF, DF, SF, NF)

Serves 4 or more

500g/18oz	Premium fat free minced beef
3	Garlic cloves, crushed (more if desired)
1 large	Onion, chopped
420g/15oz	Tomatoes, canned, chopped
1 tsp	Chili (optional)
1 tsp	Turmeric
420g/15oz	Chick peas, canned, drained
1 tbsp	Cold pressed olive oil

Heat oil in pan and brown meat. Add onion and garlic, cook for 1 minute.

Add tomatoes, chili, turmeric and simmer until meat is tender.

Stir in chick peas until heated through.

Serve with a tossed green salad.

Marsala Lamb Curry (GF, DF, SF, NF)

Serves 6

Flavor improves if made 1 - 2 days ahead and refrigerated.

2 kg/70oz	Leg of lamb boned, cubed
1/4 cup	Cold pressed olive oil
2 large	Onions, chopped
4 large	Tomatoes, chopped
1/2 cup	Water or stock
1/2 cup	Coriander, fresh, chopped

Marsala paste

Blend or process all ingredients until smooth.

1/2 cup	*Coriander, fresh*
1/2 cup	*Mint, fresh*
4	*Garlic cloves, crushed*
1 tsp	*Ginger, grated*
1/2 tsp	*Garam marsala*
1/2 tsp	*Chili, fresh, diced (optional)*
1/2 tsp	*Ground cardamom*
1/4 cup	*Apple cider vinegar*

Heat oil in large pan.

Brown single layers of lamb at a time until browned all over.

Brown onion.

Add tomatoes and blended marsala paste, cover.

Reduce heat and simmer for 45 minutes or until lamb is tender.

Serve on a bed of rice with blanched spinach and a big green salad.

Sweets, Treats and Cakes

Special Note on Using Flour

All wholemeal SR (self raising) and plain flour can be substituted with other flours. For recipes that need SR flour use 1 teaspoon of baking powder plus the other flour.

*For Gluten Free flour, a combination of buckwheat and soy flour, or rice, buckwheat and soy flour, works well. Using different flours will change the consistency of your cake or loaf, however it will still be delicious. When plain flour is needed omit the baking powder.

Banana Pops   (GF, SF)

This recipe is cool and delicious on a hot day.

Large strawberries can be prepared the same way.

2	*Passion-fruit, pulped*
1 cup	*Plain full fat yogurt*
4	*Bananas, ripe but firm*

Chopped nuts or LSA to sprinkle

Peel bananas, cut in half

Push a pop stick or bamboo skewer through center of banana

Place in freezer and freeze

Mix passion-fruit with yogurt and dip frozen banana in mixture until covered, allow to drip drain

Sprinkle with chopped nuts or LSA and return to freezer.

Healthy Treats   (GF, DF)

Each Banana

Pinch each	*Cinnamon and nutmeg*
Pinch	*Coconut shavings*
2 tsp	*Hemp seeds (optional)*

2 tsp	LSA mix – linseeds, sunflower seeds and almonds, ground
2 tsp	Raw honey
¼ tsp	70% Cocoa powder or carob powder

Grind all the seeds. Add the cinnamon and nutmeg and coconut shavings to the seeds. Place them on a plate. Skewer the banana down the middle and roll it onto the honey. Then roll the honeyed banana onto the seeds and cocoa powder.

Berry Surprise (GF, DF, NF)

Serves 4

1 cup	Raspberries, blackberries, loganberries, fresh
1 tbsp	Raw Honey OR (Cabot Health Nature Sweet Natural Sugar Substitute or Stevia may be used as a sugar substitute)
1	Orange, juiced and rind grated
2 tsp	Gelatine, dissolved in a little hot water (or agar agar)
1 cup	Plain full fat yogurt

Warm berries, honey, rind and juice. Add gelatine or agar agar mixture. Cool

Gently fold yogurt through berry mixture.

Place in 4 individual serving dishes. Chill in refrigerator.

Serve, garnished with a few extra berries and sliced kiwi fruit.

Rockmelon Pops (GF, SF)

Serves 4

1	Rockmelon
1 cup	Plain full fat dairy or coconut yogurt
1 cup	Pineapple, fresh and diced

2 tsp   *Mint, fresh, finely chopped*

Chopped nuts or LSA for sprinkles

Peel and halve and deseed the rockmelon.

Cut into wedges similar in size to half a banana.

Place a pop stick or bamboo skewer into fruit wedges.

Freeze.

Mix all these ingredients together.

Dip frozen fruit wedges into mixture until covered, allow to drip drain.

Sprinkle with chopped nuts or LSA.

Confetti Rice   (GF, DF, NF)

Serves 4

1 cup	*Coconut or almond milk*
1 tbsp	*Honey OR (Cabot Health Nature Sweet Natural Sugar Substitute or Stevia)*
1/2 cup	*Dried apricots, chopped*
1/2 cup	*Natural sultanas*
2 slices	*Mango, dried, chopped*
1.5 cups	*Rice cooked until tender*

Place fluffy rice into a saucepan with other ingredients.

Mix all together over a low heat until well combined.

If necessary, add more milk to gain your preferred consistency.

Serve warm.

Quick Mix Coconut Cake   (DF, NF)

2 cup	*Wholemeal SR flour OR (*gluten free flour)*
½ cup	*Raw sugar OR (¼ cup Cabot Health Nature Sweet Natural Sugar Substitute)*

1 cup	Coconut milk, tinned
3/4 cup	Cold pressed olive oil
3	Eggs
1 tbsp	Honey
½ cup	Coconut, shredded

Mix all ingredients in a large bowl and beat for 2 to 3 minutes, until it resembles the consistency of batter.

Pour mixture into a 23cm (9 inch) cake tin lined with baking paper.

Bake at 180C/350F for about 40 to 45 minutes - test with a skewer.

When cool sprinkle with shredded coconut.

Audrey Tea Hint

When the cake is cold cut it into 3 bars, wrap 1 or 2 bars and freeze for later. When defrosting frozen cake slice while still firm as it thaws more quickly.

Carrot and Apple Cake   (DF, SF)

1 cup	Wholemeal SF flour or (*gluten free SR flour)
1/3 cup	Honey
3/4 cup	Pecans or walnuts, chopped
1 cup	Carrot, grated
1 cup	Granny smith apple grated, leave on skin
2 tbsp	Unsweetened cocoa
1/2 tsp	Bicarb soda
2	Eggs

Sift flour, cocoa and soda into large bowl.

Mix in beaten eggs and all other ingredients and combine well.

Spoon mixture into a greased ring tin.

Bake in a moderate oven for 40 - 45 minutes or until cooked.

Test with a skewer, cool in tin.

Serve dusted with a little cinnamon.

Light and Lovely

Bananas (GF, DF, NF)

Serves 4

4 large crosswise	Bananas, peeled, sliced length ways then
1 cup	Orange juice, freshly squeezed
1/2 cup	Lemon juice, freshly squeezed
1 tbsp	Orange rind or zest
1 tbsp	Honey or Cabot Health Nature Sweet Natural Sugar Substitute
1 tsp	Cinnamon
3	Passion fruit (pulp only)

Place the juices, sweetener and rind in a large flat pan, heat until it simmers, add cinnamon, then add sliced bananas and cook for 1 to 2 minutes. Remove immediately to serving comport.

Spoon over juices and top with passion-fruit.

Tangy and Spicy Apple Bake (GF, DF, NF)

Serves 4

2 large	Green apples, peeled and cored
3 tbsp	Lemon or orange juice
1 tsp	Lemon or orange rind, grated
1 tbsp	Honey or Cabot Health Nature Sweet Natural Sugar Substitute
1 tbsp	Raisins or natural sultanas
8	Dried apricots
8	Prunes, pitted
1/2 tsp	Cinnamon, ground

Slice apples into thin wedges.

Toss in the juice.

Arrange wedges around the edge of a casserole dish.

Combine the juices with the rind, sweetener and dried fruits.

Sprinkle through the cinnamon.

Place this mixture through the center of the casserole.

Cover with foil.

Bake in a moderate oven for 30 minutes or until apple is tender.

Serve warm topped with plain full fat yogurt.

This dish can be prepared a few hours ahead, warm before serving

Orange and Coconut Cookies   (GF, DF)

1 tbsp	*Tahini*
1/4 cup	*Coconut oil, cold pressed*
½ cup	*Honey or Cabot Health Nature Sweet Natural Sugar Substitute*
1 large	*Egg, beaten*
2 tbsp	*Orange juice*
1 dstsp	*Orange rind, grated*
1.5 cups	*Stone ground wholemeal or (*Gluten free SR flour)*
1/2 cup	*Shredded coconut*
1.25 cups	*LSA – linseeds, sunflower seeds and almonds*

Mix tahini, oil and sweetener together until smooth

Stir in beaten egg, juice and rind

Add coconut, LSA and flour and combine all together

Roll teaspoonful into a ball

Flatten on tray

Bake at 180 C (350 F) for 12 - 15 minutes, until golden brown

Pear Truffles

(GF, DF)

These may be serve these with coffee after a leisurely dinner

1 cup	Pears, dried
3/4 cup	Raisins
1 tsp	Preserved ginger (more if desirable)
2 tbsp	Honey
1 tbsp	LSA – ground linseeds, sunflower seeds and almonds
1 cup	Coconut, toasted

Mince dried fruit and ginger.

Combine in a bowl with honey, LSA and 1/2 of the coconut. Mix well.

Form mixture into small balls and roll in the remaining coconut.

Slightly flatten to form thick button shapes.

Refrigerate until firm then store in fridge in an airtight container.

Can be made several days ahead.

Fruity Petit Fours

(GF, DF)

1 cup	Dried pears, chopped
1/2 cup	Dried apricots, chopped
1/2 cup	Cashews, chopped
1/2 cup	Shredded coconut
1 tbsp	Lemon juice
1 tbsp	Honey OR (Cabot Health Nature Sweet Natural Sugar Substitute)
425ml/15oz	Coconut cream

Mix all ingredients together with enough coconut cream to bind the mixture.

Stand covered for 1 hour.

If mixture is too dry add more coconut cream to hold it together and make it pliable.

Roll into small balls,

Press a cashew nut into the top of each ball.

Place in small confectionery paper patty cups.

Cover and store in fridge in an airtight container.

Fruit and Nut Salad (GF, DF, SF)

Serves 6 - 8

1	*Red apple diced, skin on, core out*
1	*Green apple diced, skin on, core out*
1 cup	*Celery, diced*
1	*Avocado diced, skin off, stone out*
425g/15oz	*Fresh pineapple or use unsweetened pineapple pieces, retain juice,*
½ cup	*Mint, finely chopped*
1 cup	*Pecans or walnuts, chopped*

Gently toss the apples and avocado in pineapple juice, drain.

Mix with all other ingredients.

Dress with no 3 dressing (see page 173)

Peachy Treats (GF, SF, NF)

Serves 6 to 8

Made in a flash, this dessert is light and very tasty.

Peach or pear halves can be used.

825g/30oz	*Peach halves, drained or 6 - 8 fresh peaches*
100g/3-4oz	*Plain full fat yogurt*
1 cup	*Mixed dried fruit, chopped*
1 tbsp	*Apple or orange juice*

1 pinch	Ground cinnamon
1/2 cup	Toasted coconut

Arrange peach halves in individual serving dishes.

Mix fruit juice with dried fruit.

Stand for about 1/2 hour, then fold into yogurt.

Spoon mixture into hollows of peaches, sprinkle with cinnamon.

Top each serve with coconut.

Basic Gluten Free Pastry (GF, DF, SF, NF)

2 tbsp	Gelatine or agar agar
1/2 tsp	Bicarbonate soda
1/2 cup	Water
1/2 cup	Cold pressed olive oil
1/2 tsp	Salt
1/2	Lemon, juiced
200g/7oz	Potato and chick pea flour
50g/2oz	Rice flour
50g/2oz	Arrowroot

Preheat the oven to 180C/350F.

Dissolve gelatine in hot water.

Put gelatine, lemon and oil into a large ceramic bowl.

Sift flours, salt and bicarb into the oil and gelatine mixture.

Mix the dough until it pulls away from the side and forms a ball.

Take two pieces of plastic or cling wrap.

Place one piece of plastic wrap on a board or a clean surface you wish to roll the dough on.

Place the ball of dough onto the board and then place the second piece of plastic wrap on top of the dough.

Roll out between these 2 sheets of plastic, to desired thickness, then discard plastic wrap.

When handling the dough, rub a small amount of oil on your hands.

Bake in the oven for approx 15 minutes, until golden brown

Goodness Cake (DF, SF)

This cake is unbelievably tasty, nutritious and energy boosting. Store in an airtight container.

1 cup	Natural sultanas
1 cup	Medjool dates, chopped
1 cup	Dried apricots, chopped
1 cup	Brazil nuts, chopped
1 cup	Sunflower seeds
1/4 cup	LSA (linseeds, sunflower seeds and almonds – ground) or hemp seeds
1/4 cup	Sesame seeds
1 tsp	Mixed spice
2	Eggs, beaten
2 cups	Wholemeal SR flour OR (*Gluten free SR flour)
2 cups	Orange juice, fresh

Place all ingredients, except the flour and eggs, into a large saucepan. Bring slowly to the boil, stirring continually. Simmer for 3 to 5 minutes.

Cool, then stir in eggs and flour.

Grease and line a cake tin then place the mixture into the lined tin.

Bake in a slow oven at about 150C/300F for 1 hour or until cooked, when tested with a skewer.

Cool cake in the tin.

Hint to Make Nut Milk

To make one cup of nut milk mix one cup of hot water or fruit juice with two tablespoons of any nut butter such as hazel nut, Brazil nut, cashew nut, or almond and mix in a blender until smooth.

Carob Fruit Loaf   (DF, SF)

1 cup	Mixed dried fruit
1 cup	Wheat germ or LSA – ground linseeds, sunflower seeds and almonds
1.5 cups	Rice milk or coconut milk
1/4 cup	Carob powder
1 cup	Wholemeal SF flour OR (*Gluten free SR flour)

Place fruit, wheat germ or LSA and milk in a large bowl.

Cover and let stand for 2 hours.

Fold in sifted carob and flour and mix well.

Place in lined loaf tin and bake at 180C/350F for 45 to 60 minutes.

Cool cake in the tin.

Banana Cake   (GF*, NF)

250g/9oz	Wholemeal SR flour OR (*gluten free SR flour)
1/2 cup	Cold pressed olive or coconut oil
125g/4-5oz	Honey or Naturesweet Sugar Substitute
2 large	Ripe bananas, mashed
3 tbsp	Milk or rice milk
1 tsp	Bicarb soda
1 tsp	Vanilla
2	Eggs

Beat oil and sugar until smooth.

Add eggs, beat well.

Add mashed bananas, mix in the milk, bicarb soda and vanilla.

Add alternately with sifted flour until all ingredients are folded smoothly together.

Place mixture in a lined cake tin.

Sprinkled with cinnamon or chopped walnuts.

Cook in a moderate oven for about 45 minutes, test with skewer.

Cool in tin for 10 minutes before removing to a cooling rack.

Poached Fruitee Pears   (GF, DF)

Serves 4 or more

3 large	*Pears, peeled and cored*
1/2 cup	*Dried apricots, chopped*
1/2 cup	*Shredded coconut*
1/4 cup	*Almonds, chopped*
1/2 tsp	*Cinnamon*
1 tsp	*Honey (more if desired)*
1 cup	*Apple or apricot juice*

Cut pears in half and lay center-up in a casserole dish.

In a bowl mix together apricots, coconut, almonds and cinnamon.

Add enough honey to bind the mixture together.

Divide the mixture evenly over the six pear halves.

Add one cup of juice to casserole, pour gently over the fruit.

Cover and bake in preheated oven at 180C/350F for approx 30 minutes.

Serve barely warm, with frozen apple and pear dessert.

Apple and Pear Ice Cream   (GF)

Serves 4

1	*Pear, stem removed, skin on*
1	*Granny smith apple, skin on*

3	Passion-fruit pulp
1/2 cup	Milk or plain full fat yogurt
1 tsp	Honey or Naturesweet Sugar Substitute
1 tbsp	Gelatine, or agar agar
425ml/15oz	Coconut cream or dairy cream

Mix all ingredients together in a food processor until smooth.

Pour into a container of your choice and freeze.

Serve in scoops with crushed almonds or with poached pears.

The following recipe is a very special Christmas Treat using fabulous, raw, healthy and very delicious ingredients. Recipe from nutritionist Kylie McCarthy

White Choc Cherry Cheese Cake   (GF, DF)

Makes 12 servings, Soak time: 2 hours, Prep time: 45mins

Chill Time: 2 hours

This classic cheesecake will make anyone want to go raw. The crunchy, salted texture of the crust, the creamy cake, and the sweet, tart cherries make this one of the superstar desserts in my collection.

Crust

225g	Walnuts, soaked 6-8 hrs and dehydrated (If you do not have a dehydrator, place them in the oven on a tray -on really low heat (50deg) for 1/2 an hour. Keep an eye on them - ovens vary.)
1/3 cup (48g)	Medjool dates
1/4 cup (30g)	Palm sugar
1/4 cup (20g)	Cacao powder
1/4 cup (44g)	Cacao nibs
1/8 teaspoon	sea salt

Filling

3 cups (360g)	*Cashews, soaked 2 hours*
1 cup (235m)	*Basic nut milk - if you don't want to make your own nut milk, bought Almond milk is OK.*
3/4 cup (255g)	*Honey or Agave nectar*
1/4 cup (60ml)	*Lemon juice*
2 tbsp (30ml)	*Organic vanilla extract*
1/4 cup (30g)	*Lecithin powder - Sunflower lecithin is a better choice as most lecithin is made of soy. Soy products are genetically modified (alarm bells) so source yourself sunflower lecithin.*
3/4 cup (164g)	*Cacao butter, warmed to liquid*

Topping

2 cups (310g)	*Fresh or frozen cherries, pitted and thawed.*

Method - Crust

In a food processor, grind the walnuts into a flour.

Add the dates and palm sugar and process until incorporated.

Add the cacao powder, cacao nibs, and sea salt and process again until the mixture starts to stick together.

Reserve 1/4 cup (60g) of the crust for the topping.

Spread the mixture evenly into a 9 inch (23cm) spring form pan lined with baking paper.

Starting in the center, press the mixture firmly and work your way out.

Make the crust as even as possible. Don't forget the edges.

Method - Filling

Place the cashews, nut milk, agave, lemon juice, and vanilla into a high power blender and process until very smooth. Add the lecithin and cacao butter and blend again.

Pour the filling onto the crust.

Smooth using an offset spatula.

Spread 1 cup (155g) of the cherries over the top of the filing, staggering them evenly.

Use a toothpick to gently push the cherries into the filling. Alternatively, you can spread the cherries over the crust and pour the filling over them. I prefer to place them myself so I have an evenly polka-dotted cheesecake.

Spread the remaining cherries over the top in the empty areas. Gently press the cherries half way down into the mixture with your finger.

Sprinkle the reserved crust mix lightly over the top

Place the cheesecake straight in the freezer for 2 hours. Let thaw before serving.

The Almond pulp from your home made Almond Milk can be popped into the freezer to be used as a base to your grain free slices or biscuits- YUMMO! ha!

Store in the freezer for 1 month or in the refrigerator for 3 days.

Variation: *Substitute your favorite berries in place of cherries.*

Appendix

Conversion Chart for Recipes and Cooking

Ounces	Grams
1	28
2	57
3	85
4	113
5	142
6	170
7	198
8	227
9	255
10	283

For additional amounts select the appropriate conversion above and multiply or add or both.

For example 15 ounces = 10 ounces (283 grams)

+ 5 ounces (142 grams) = 15 ounces (425 grams)

Pounds	Kilograms
1	0.45
2	0.91
3	1.36
4	1.81
5	2.27
6	2.72
7	3.17
8	3.63
9	4.10

Pounds	Kilograms
10	4.54

Temperature Fahrenheit	Temperature Centigrade
200	93
250	121
300	149
350	177
400	204

For other temperature conversions use the following formula:

F to C : subtract 32, then divide by 1.8

C to F : multiply by 1.8, then add 32

Kitchen Measures

Measure	Ounces	Milliliters
One teaspoon	0.17	5
One tablespoon	0.5	14
One cup	8	227
One pint	16	454
One quart	32	908
One gallon	128	3632

Helpful Conversions

Ounces to milliliters: multiply ounce figure by 30 to get number of milliliters

Pounds to kilograms: multiply pound figure by 0.45 to get number of kilograms

Pounds to grams: multiply pound figure by 453 to get number of grams

Grams to ounces: multiply gram figure by .0353 to get number of ounces

Ounces to grams: multiply ounce figure by 28.3 to get number of grams

One teaspoon = 5 grams

Three teaspoons = one tablespoon =1/2 ounce = 14.3 grams

Two tablespoons = one ounce = 28.35 grams

Agar-agar (1 bar) = 4-6 tablespoons agar-agar flakes

Garlic concentrated (1 teaspoon) = 2 cloves fresh garlic

Herbs, dried (1/2 teaspoon) = 2 tablespoons fresh herbs

Sweeteners Equivalents

1/2 cup sweetener	1/2 cup maple syrup
	1/2 cup coconut sugar
	1/2 cup raw sugar
	1/3 cup molasses
	1/2 cup honey
	1+1/2 cups barley malt extract
	1/2 cup fruit juice concentrate
	1/2 cup fruit juice
	1/2 cup unsweetened frozen juice concentrate
	1/3 cup Nature Sweet Sugar Substitute

Quick Bowel Cleanse and Detox

Why Cleanse the Bowel ?

A good cleansing program should always begin by removing the waste in your colon, which is the last portion of your food processing chain. If you attempt to clean your liver or blood stream without addressing a bowel filled with toxic waste material, some of the toxins excreted in your bile will probably get recycled back to your liver and lymphatic system.

It is vital to remove waste and toxins from the colon and we need to understand the importance of frequent, easily passed bowel movements. Gastroenterologist, Dr. Anthony Bassler, tells his colleagues, "Every physician should realize that intestinal toxemias (poisons) are the most important contributing causes of many disorders and the diseases of the human body."

Waste products, bad bacteria and old feces that linger too long in the colon cause inflammation in the lining of the colon; if chronic, this inflammation may cause bowel polyps and cancers to form.

Once your small and large intestines are clean you will be able to absorb nutrients efficiently again! This will produce more energy and a sense of general well-being after cleaning your bowel. The major part of the body's supply of serotonin (the good mood chemical) is manufactured in your intestines. By cleaning the toxins and old fecal matter out of your colon your mood will improve, as you will be able to synthesize serotonin more efficiently!

You need to drink lots of water while doing a bowel cleanse and warm water is preferable. The warm water will stimulate the muscular contractions of the intestines (peristalsis); whereas cold water is not as effective at this. Drink at least 70 ounces (2 liters) of water a day.

Observe your bowel actions

Always have a look at your bowel actions to observe their color and consistency. Your bowel actions can be very light brown to dark brown or greenish in color, which is all normal. If your bowel actions are black (similar to a black tar color) this is abnormal and may indicate bleeding from the bowel. If there is red blood in your feces, this also indicates bleeding from the bowel or from hemorrhoids. Always tell your doctor, as this can be a sign of bowel cancer. Many people will find the idea of checking their bowel actions a little gross or distasteful. But if you can't see what you're eliminating, then you can't see the results!

Things you may find in your bowel actions-

Mucoid plaque is the old putrefied fecal matter that has been stuck to the sides and corners of your colon and small intestine. This may have been stuck in your bowel for months all the while causing inflammation and reducing the absorption of nutrients. See page 265

Quick Detox Diet

One to two week Bowel Cleansing Diet

During your bowel cleanse try to improve your diet as per the following:

Prohibited Foods to Avoid on Your Detox

- Sugar and foods containing added sugar
- Deep fried foods, but you can have stir fries with cold pressed olive oil
- All red meats, pork, poultry and all preserved meats such as bacon, jerky, salami and smoked meats and smoked fish.
- All alcohol
- Coffee and tea (except herbal tea)
- All dairy products – cheese, butter, margarine, ice cream, and cream and dairy milk
- Fast foods and processed foods such as donuts, pretzels, fries, etc

If you are gluten intolerant, please avoid gluten containing foods such as wheat, rye, barley and oats. During a bowel cleanse whole corn, lentils and quinoa are preferable to gluten containing grains.

For some people, even those who are not gluten intolerant, a better bowel cleanse is achieved if all grains are eliminated during the detox period.

Only these foods are allowed on your detox

• Raw salads made with all types of lettuce, radicchio, cabbage, rocket, cucumber, capsicums (bell peppers), celery, walnuts, hemp seeds, apples, olives, avocado, tomatoes and carrots. Try to include some red radish, onions, garlic, ginger, oregano, parsley, cilantro and basil, as these are natural antibiotics. You can use a grater or a garlic crush or a machine which chops things very finely. Grating hard vegetables makes them easier to digest.

• Cooked vegetables of ALL varieties; you can have these vegetables roasted, baked, stir fried, steamed or in a vegetable soup. To flavor the soup you may use miso, Herbamare salt, sea salt, pepper and/or vegetable stock. Garlic, onions and radishes are excellent bowel cleansers and can be eaten cooked and raw.

• Raw fruits and stewed fruits – berries, apples, stone fruits, pears, kiwi, banana, and citrus fruits. If desired, stew the fruits in their own juice with stevia or Nature Sweet Sugar Substitute. Make sure the fruits are not moldy and are washed to remove contaminants.

• Oils – allowed oils to use are cold pressed olive oil, coconut oil and macadamia oils.

• Milks – allowed milks are coconut milk, rice milk or almond milk

• Raw nuts and seeds are allowed – these include Brazil nuts, almonds, cashews, walnuts, hazel nuts, ground flaxseeds, LSA, hemp seeds, chia seeds and pumpkin seeds. You can grind the seeds in a coffee grinder or food processor.

• Tahini and hummus may be eaten and are excellent for the digestive system and provide easily absorbed minerals especially calcium.

• Salad dressings – allowed ingredients are cold pressed olive oil, organic apple cider vinegar, fresh lemon or lime juice, mustard, hummus and tahini.

- Raw juices made with carrot, apple, cabbage, kale, lime, orange, grapefruit, lemon, and mint can help to heal the gut and reduce parasites. You do not have to include all of these at one time if your digestive system is sensitive just start with 3 or 4 ingredients. A dash of the fresh herbs oregano, thyme or coriander (cilantro) add more potent antibiotic effects.. You can freeze the juices immediately after making them and store them in containers in the freezer. If you freeze them immediately after making them this will retain all the healing properties of the juices. This enables you to avoid cleaning the juicer every day. During a bowel cleanse you can drink approximately 200 to 400 mls (7 to 12 ounces) of juice daily. If the juice is too strong in flavor or effect you can dilute it with water or extra apple and carrot.

Supplements to take during your bowel cleanse:

FiberTone powder is a suitable gluten free fiber to use during the detox. Mix the FiberTone powder in 180mls (6 ounces) of water, raw juice or a smoothie. You can also add FiberTone to a mixture of ground seeds and nuts. FiberTone is very high in fiber and can be safely taken long term to support stronger bowel function.

Glutamine Powder - Glutamine supports healthy bowel function and the repair of bowel inflammation caused from many injurious factors such as - unfriendly bacteria, parasites, steroid drugs, antibiotic drugs and autoimmune dysfunction. Glutamine powder is best taken for several months after your bowel cleanse is finished. Take a dose of one tsp of glutamine powder once or twice daily. Take glutamine with cold or room temperature liquids. Glutamine should not be added to hot beverages because heat damages it.

LivaTone Plus which contains Milk Thistle, Selenium, Taurine, B and C vitamins, N-Acetyl-Cysteine and antioxidants.

Detox Notes:

- During your bowel cleanse, you do not have to eat anything that you do not enjoy or anything that upsets your digestive system. Avoid things that you are allergic to.

- Do not cook with a microwave oven during your detox, as this will irradiate your food.

Fermented Foods

Fermented foods are a potent way to use food to increase the quantity and diversity of beneficial bacterial species inhabiting our digestive system.

Normal gut flora has more than 500 different species and most available commercial probiotic products contain a maximum of nine species. Fermented foods contain trillions of beneficial bacteria compared to probiotic supplements which are limited to billions. Furthermore, fermented foods have a wider variety of beneficial bacterial species compared to probiotic supplements. They are also generally more cost effective.

After any course of antibiotics it is necessary to repopulate our intestine with as wide a variety of micro-organisms as possible.

Fermented foods such as sauerkraut, blue cheese and natto (a soy dish popular in Japan), contain substantial amounts of vitamin K2. Natto contains the highest concentration of K2 of any food measured; nearly all of it is present as MK-7, which research has shown to be a highly effective form. Vitamin K2 helps prevent osteoporosis and fights some types of cancer.

Fermented Dairy Products

Yogurt – purchase full fat, unsweetened, unflavored and preferably organic or biodynamic.

Yogurt may be made at home either by using prepared yogurt as a starter or a commercial product like EasyYo or Progurt may be used. Avoid the sweetened choices.

Kefir – is a cultured milk; it's easy to make at home from either commercially available freeze dried granules or working grains to convert milk proteins from hard to easy to digest.

Cheese

Camembert, Brie, moldy cheeses – always buy these fresh, and do not allow them to age for too long.

Buttermilk – most commercial buttermilk is not cultured but a soured version of this wonderful food, which tastes like drinking yogurt, is available.

Crème fraiche - is cultured cream. The product is churned, resulting in butter and buttermilk being separated.

Fermented Vegetable Products

Sauerkraut – is a traditional European winter food. It is traditionally cabbage based with other available vegetables added, salted and naturally fermented with fresh liquid whey from either aged yogurt or kefir.

Kalekraut – is very similar to Sauerkraut but is made with kale instead of cabbage. It is made the same way and the resultant product tends to be less sour in flavor.

Kim Chi – is the national dish of Korea and is made in a similar way to sauerkraut with the addition of many other vegetables, spices and especially chili. It also tends to be highly salted and many have added salted fish.

Fermented Grains

Sourdough bread – by definition this bread uses wild yeasts to effect the fermentation. It is best to rotate production and aim for a 3 day turnaround for each batch. Unfortunately most commercially available products are based on a 24 hour batch time and this is insufficient time to denature the gluten in the bread dough. If you are gluten intolerant, avoid breads with gluten containing grains.

Fermented Soy

Natto – definitely not for the faint hearted. This food is eaten with gusto in Japan but in western countries it has not gained the same popularity. Natto is soy beans that have been fermented with a bacteria and the product is distinctive.

Miso – is a mash of soy, barley or rice or a mixture of these, which is fermented with a beneficial fungus. Miso can be mixed with water and tofu as a soup, or may be added to meals to impart flavor and beneficial nutrients.

Tempeh - is very similar to miso but the beneficial fungus is grown on whole soybeans and is eaten in a similar way to tofu.

Fermented Teas and Fruits

Kombucha – this requires sweetened tea for the growth of this probiotic rich drink. It is made by adding a bought 'scoby' to cooled and sweetened tea. It is then left to ferment at room temperature until sweetness is replaced by a more acidic taste.

Apple cider vinegar – for its probiotic value it is best to buy an organic brand with a "mother" in it. The mother is cloudy sediment on the bottom of the bottle, and this provides a rich source of probiotics.

Vinegar is probably our best known household fermented food and it produced from further fermentation of wines, fruit or flowers that have been used to produce alcohol. Inferior vinegars are simply diluted acetic acid and are definitely not a healthy alternative.

NOTE: This list is not exhaustive. There are many more varieties.

Eating Liver as food

The liver of mammals and poultry are commonly eaten as food by humans. Domestic pig, ox, lamb, calf, chicken, and goose livers are widely available from butchers and supermarkets.

In general, organ meats are much higher in nutrients than muscle meats.

Remember that vegetables and fruits are rich in anti-inflammatory and anti-cancer phyto-nutrients that are not present in high concentrations in any meats, including organ meats, so fresh plant food should always be a large part of your diet.

A popular objection to eating liver is the belief that the liver is the storage organ for toxins in the body. While it is true that the liver neutralizes toxins (such as medicines, chemical agents and poisons), it does NOT store these toxins. Toxins that the body cannot eliminate accumulate in the body's fatty tissues such as the endocrine and nervous systems.

The liver is a storage organ for vitally important nutrients (vitamins A, D, E, K, B 12, folic acid, copper and iron). These nutrients provide the body with some of the tools it needs to get rid of toxins.

It is far healthier to eat muscle meats and organ meats from animals that have been raised on fresh pastures and not given hormones, antibiotics or commercial feed. Pasture-raised animal meats and milks are much higher in nutrients than animal products that come from commercial feedlots. Meat from pasture-raised animals has 2 to 4 times more omega-3 fatty acids than meat from commercially-raised animals.

Eggs from pasture fed chickens have been shown to contain up to 19 times more omega-3 fatty acids than supermarket eggs! In addition to these nutritional advantages, pasture-raised animal products benefit local farmers and communities as well as the environment.

Preparing your food

You may spend time, money and effort sourcing healthy and/ or organic food but if you do not prepare or cook it in a healthy manner, you will not gain the benefits to your health

Eating most of your food in its raw state is ideal, however most busy people are not going to be able to accomplish a completely raw diet, and we'll end up cooking some of our food.

Wise food preparation starts with high quality whole (preferably organic and/or locally grown) foods and food preparation from scratch. It takes more time of course, but just look at the benefits to your health and longevity. Bowel cancer rates are soaring and digestive disorders are epidemic, and poor food preparation and cooking methods are partly to blame. I am against the use of microwave ovens to cook and reheat food and we really should be wondering why bowel cancer rates have increased dramatically since the introduction of microwave ovens.

Now if you want to sterilize a dishcloth or heat a cup of coffee then use your microwave. Reserve its use for cleaning tea towels, dishrags and sponges. Wet these things first and then heat them for two minutes on high; they are great at effectively sterilizing these often dirty and contaminated sources of bacteria. But if you zap your food in a microwave you are compromising your health.

Alternatives to using a microwave oven include -

- Stir fry your food in a wok

- Roast your meat and vegetables in a traditional oven

- Purchase a turbo oven, which is economical and a healthy way to cook or reheat leftovers. The turbo oven allows you to make meals in half the time of traditional ovens

- A convection oven is an easy way to reheat leftovers. Use them at a low temperature — like 200-250 degrees F — to warm a meal over 20-30 minutes

- Try to eat more of your food in its raw state, as it gives you maximum nutritional value and contains living enzymes and probiotics

- Prepare your meals in advance. This way you will always have a healthy meal available on those days when you're too busy to cook. Make soups and casseroles in bulk, and then freeze them in large freezer bags or glass jars. Before mealtime, just take one out and defrost it in a sink of warm water. Slowly reheat your meal on the stove-top.

Microwave ovens are super convenient but they are bad for your food, and bad for your health.

The health concerns with microwave ovens include:

- Cancer causing toxins can be leached into your food from plastic or paper covers, wrappings or plates during heating.

- The food temperature may become extremely hot; this can cause burns or steam buildup that could explode--this is especially bad for baby bottles, and is one of the reasons why baby bottles should NEVER be heated in the microwave. Microwave heating can destroy the disease-fighting ability of breast milk or milk with added probiotics.

- Plant foods and other foods lose phyto-nutrients, which fight and prevent cancer when cooked in the microwave.

- The microwave generated heat produces extremely rapid vibration of the molecules in the cell structures in food so that the physical and chemical structure of foods change; the long term effects are unknown.

- Microwave radiation leakage—microwave ovens vary in the amount of radiation that escapes while they are in use. But even if your microwave is in top condition, be aware that standing a foot away from it while it's running can expose you to upwards of 400 milliGauss, and a mere 4 milliGauss has been linked to leukemia.

There have been insufficient studies done to determine what types of damage occur in foods during microwaving, and I think this is because there is not enough to be gained financially from such research. In 1991 there was a legal case involving a woman who had hip surgery and died because the blood used in her blood transfusion was warmed in a microwave oven. Blood is routinely warmed before transfusions, but not by microwave. The microwave altered the blood in such a profound way that it caused her death.

Microwave cooking vibrates the molecules in your food to levels they were never designed to experience in nature. This tends to damage the fragile nutrients in ways we do not fully understand – so why are so many people willing to be guinea pigs – or perhaps we are just way too trusting of common day practices?

Let's look at some of the research available:

- A 1999 Scandinavian study of the cooking of asparagus spears found that microwaving caused a reduction in vitamin C.

- Microwaving can destroy the essential disease-fighting substances in breast milk. In 1992, Quan found that microwaved breast milk lost lysozyme activity and antibodies, and fostered the growth of more potentially pathogenic bacteria.

- In a study of the super food garlic, as little as 60 seconds of microwave heating was sufficient to inactivate its allinase, which is garlic's principle active ingredient against cancer.

- A Japanese study by Watanabe showed that just 6 minutes of microwave heating turned a large percentage of the Vitamin B12 in milk into a useless form.

- A 2008 Australian study showed that microwaves cause a higher degree of "protein unfolding" than conventional heating. This means proteins are damaged.

- A study published in the November 2003 issue of The Journal of the Science of Food and Agriculture found that broccoli "zapped" in the microwave lost up to 97 percent of its antioxidants. By comparison, steamed broccoli lost only 11 percent or fewer of its antioxidants. There were also reductions in beneficial phenolic compounds and glucosinolates, but mineral levels remained intact.

To me this is very worrying and enough reason to stop using your microwave oven. However there are still more unknown dangers, because as well as the loss of nutrients, microwaving forms new compounds (known as radiolytic compounds). These compounds are foreign to humans and nature, and we do not know their effects in the human body.

Dr. Hans Hertel, a Swiss food scientist, found negative effects in human blood tests from using microwave cooking. Dr Hertel did a small but high-quality study which showed that microwave cooking altered the food's nutrients enough to cause changes in the subject's blood and these changes appeared negative.

The changes included:

• Increased cholesterol levels

• Decreased numbers of leukocytes (white blood cells)

• Decreased numbers of red blood cells

• Production of radiolytic compounds (compounds unknown in nature)

• Decreased hemoglobin levels, which could indicate anemic tendencies

Dr. Hertel and his team published the results in 1992, but a Swiss trade organization, the Swiss Association of Dealers for Electro-apparatuses for Households and Industry, had a gag order issued, which prohibited Dr. Hertel from declaring that microwaves were dangerous to health. The gag order was later removed in 1998, after the Swiss court ruled that the gag order violated the right to freedom of expression.

Aloe Vera

How to make your own gel

Most species of aloe are useful for both internal and external use. The only considerations are if you are sensitive to the active chemicals found in the yellow layer found just under the skin of the plant.

Plants attain their medicinal value after 3 years so it is best to buy a mature plant. As the plant matures it assumes a more rounded leaf pattern and flowers after two to three years.

Aloe Vera

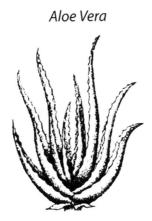

Unflavored aloe juice is available commercially but it is so easy to produce the product yourself with a kitchen blender.

To make your own aloe vera gel (juice) simply take approximately 1/3 of a mature leaf and wash it to remove dust and pollution. Remove the spines from the side of the leaf and cut it into smaller chunks and blend in your blender/food processor. When completely liquidized add it to your fresh low sugar vegetable juice or water and enjoy.

Aloe vera gel alkalizes the body and protects and soothes the intestinal lining. This can provide relief from gastritis, acid stomach, reflux and heartburn and gastric ulcers. It can also soothe and protect an inflamed colon. It can reduce constipation and irritable bowel syndrome. Aloe vera inhibits the growth of detrimental bacteria and yeasts and is a valuable prebiotic for beneficial bacteria.

Tests for Bowel and Digestive Function

If you believe that you may have a digestive or bowel problem it is a good idea to see a specialist in gastrointestinal disorders; such a specialist is known as a gastroenterologist. A gastroenterologist will take an extensive history of your symptoms and bowel actions. The most serious problems to exclude are malignant tumors of the stomach and bowels, which become far more common as we age. This is why it is important to have thorough investigations early on, if you develop any change in bowel actions, unexplained weight loss or abdominal pains.

Complete Diagnostic Stool Analysis (CDSA)

Specialized tests known as a "Complete Diagnostic Stool Analysis" (CDSA) can be done by doctors and naturopaths interested in nutritional medicine.

The CDSA is divided into panel A and panel B.

Panel A assesses the overall appearance of your bowel actions (stools), as well as checking them for blood cells and fat globules. It also measures the stools for markers of food digestion and absorption, such as triglyceride fats, chymotrypsin enzyme, meat fibers, vegetable cells and fibers, acid-base balance, and short chain fatty acids such as valerate and iso-butyrate, long chain fatty acids, cholesterol and total fecal fat. Panel A will give your doctor a very good evaluation of your ability to digest and absorb a wide range of food groups. This is important because even though you may have an excellent diet, you may not be able to extract the vital nutrients from your food if your liver, gallbladder, pancreas, stomach or intestines are malfunctioning.

Panel B assesses the types and amounts of microorganisms in your gut. This is done using microscopy and cultures to look for parasites, bacteria and fungi.

It is also possible to test for a common stomach bacteria called Helicobacter pylori, which is the cause of gastric and duodenal ulcers. Testing for the Helicobacter Direct Antigen in the stools can do this.

Bristol Stool Chart

	Type 1	Separate hard lumps	Very constipated
	Type 2	Lumpy and sausage like	Slightly constipated
	Type 3	A sausage shape with cracks in the surface	Normal
	Type 4	Like a smooth, soft sausage or snake	Normal
	Type 5	Soft blobs with clear-cut edges	Lacking fiber
	Type 6	Mushy consistency with ragged edges	Inflammation
	Type 7	Liquid consistency with no solid pieces	Inflammation

Things you may find in your bowel actions

Mucoid plaque is the old putrefied fecal matter that has been stuck to the sides and corners of your colon and small intestine. This may have been stuck in your bowel for months, all the while causing inflammation and reducing the absorption of nutrients.

Mucoid plaque forming foods are: sugar, processed foods, refined flour and preserved meat. Mucoid plaque has different shapes and sizes depending from which area in your gut it originated. It may resemble ropes; these are discs and balls held together by stringy mucus like substances. These ropes can get quite long and their color may vary from yellow-green, light brown to very dark brown. They should not be tar black, as this indicates bleeding from the bowel, which is often a sign of bowel cancer. Mucoid plaque can look quite weird and may be soft, firm or rubbery. If you have ever had a colonic irrigation (professional enema) you may have eliminated this rubbery old fecal matter out of your bowels before.

Mucoid plaque

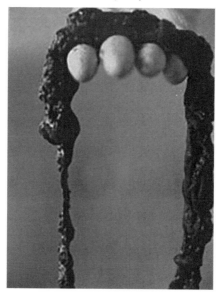

Some of my patients have passed strange looking objects or worms and that's why it's important to check your bowel actions during a bowel cleanse. If you do pass anything that moves, such as a worm, keep it in a jar for you doctor to check at the lab.

Colonoscopy

This involves passing a thin flexible fiber-optic tube called a colonoscope through the anus. This procedure enables the doctor to visualize the lining of the entire colon and rectum, and transmits the picture to a television screen. Samples (biopsies) can be taken from suspicious looking areas of the bowel to enable accurate diagnosis. It is done under mild intravenous sedation and takes around 30 minutes. The test is usually not uncomfortable. The colon needs to be cleansed with laxatives beforehand to enable an accurate assessment. Colonoscopy is the most accurate way to diagnose the cause of bowel symptoms and to screen for cancer and bowel polyps. Bowel polyps can be removed via this procedure. There is a slight risk of perforation of the colon (1 in 2000 cases) during colonoscopy.

Colonoscopy

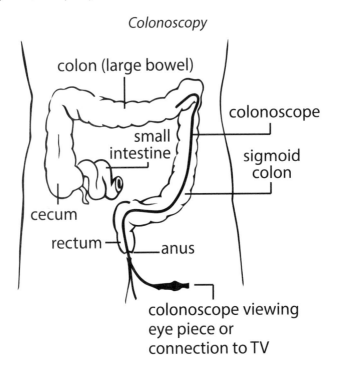

Sigmoidoscopy

This is similar to colonoscopy, however the tube that is passed up into the bowel is much shorter and can only assess the lower part of the large bowel (rectum and sigmoid colon). It is usually done in your doctor's office. This test takes around 5 minutes and may cause a feeling of gas and slight cramping. An enema is required to cleanse the bowel beforehand.

Small Bowel Capsule Endoscopy

We live in an amazing world where medicine has enabled the small intestinal lining to be examined by a video camera inside a capsule which is swallowed by the patient.

The SmartPill is a small camera inside a capsule which is swallowed and moves through the entire digestive tract, sending information back to a cell-phone-sized receiver worn around the person's waist.

The endoscope is a vitamin-pill sized capsule equipped with its own camera and light source. While the video capsule passes through the digestive tract, images are transmitted to a data recorder worn on a waist belt. After the procedure, the doctor views a color video taken from the capsule.

This capsule examines the three portions (duodenum, jejunum and ileum) of a patient's small intestine. The video capsule camera can identify different abnormalities present within the small intestine. It has become an important tool for diagnosis of suspected diseases in the small bowel.

Capsule endoscopy is useful for diagnosing diseases in the small intestine, and can sometimes find sources of occult bleeding (microscopic bleeding not seen by the naked eye). It can diagnose causes of abdominal pain such as stomach and duodenal ulcers, cancer and Crohn's disease. Although capsule endoscopy can be used to diagnose problems in the small intestine, unlike colonoscopy it cannot treat problems that may be discovered. A radio-frequency signal can be used to accurately estimate the location of the capsule and to track it in real time inside the intestines.

Common reasons for doing capsule endoscopy include unexplained bleeding, unexplained iron deficiency, unexplained abdominal pain, search for polyps, ulcers and tumors of small intestine and inflammatory bowel disease such as Crohn's disease

Preparation for Capsule Endoscopy

Patients fast the day before the procedure, as an empty stomach allows optimal viewing conditions. You should inform the doctor of any medications you take, the presence of a pacemaker, previous abdominal surgery, swallowing problems or previous history of obstructions in the bowel. After ingesting the capsule and until it is excreted, patients should not have a Magnetic Resonance Imaging (MRI) examination or be near an MRI device.

The capsule is disposable and progresses naturally with your bowel movement and is eliminated with a bowel action. It does not need to be recovered from your bowel actions. There is not any pain or discomfort during capsule excretion. It is a very safe procedure because a capsule endoscopy does not require sedation and air insufflations and thus eliminates the risks associated with sedation and perforation of the bowel which can occur during conventional endoscopy. The capsule is single use, which diminishes the risk of infection acquired from reprocessing surgical equipment.

Rarely there is retention of the capsule. It is important for you to inform your doctor if you experience signs of possible complications, such as fever and vomiting, trouble swallowing, chest or abdominal pain or vomiting.

Ultrasound Scans

Ultrasound uses a transducer to bounce painless sound waves off organs to create an image of their structure. This is a safe procedure and does not involve any radiation. The ultrasound images can show up diseases of the gallbladder disease, liver, spleen and pancreas.

Barium Enema X-ray

This is an X-ray examination of the large bowel (rectum and colon) which enables the doctor to assess the shape, size and smoothness of the outline of your large bowel. The X-ray is performed after you receive an enema to insert barium (a chalky radio-opaque liquid) into the rectum. The barium will contrast and outline the wall of the large bowel. A barium enema will show up enlargement of the large bowel and irregularities of the bowel wall and bowel pockets known as diverticula. It can also reveal muscular spasm (spastic colon) in the wall of the large bowel.

In some cases of severe constipation a barium enema X-ray will reveal a huge dilated colon with extra loops of bowel (redundant bowel); this is known as a "megacolon".

A barium enema may show some types of bowel cancer, however it can also miss many small cancers, and for this reason a colonoscopy is a far more accurate way to exclude bowel cancer.

The upper intestines, namely the esophagus and stomach and duodenum can be visualized with a barium X-ray. The patient is given a drink containing radio-opaque barium and this can show problems with swallowing, obstructions in the esophagus, a sliding hiatus hernia, reflux and stomach tumors etc.

Stomach acid test

The stomach acid test is used to measure the amount of acid and the level of acidity in the stomach contents. This test is known as the gastric acid secretion test.

The stomach contents are removed through a tube that is passed into the stomach through the mouth and then into the esophagus. The stomach contents are analyzed for the amount and concentration of acid in a laboratory.

The hormone gastrin may be injected into your body to stimulate the stomach cells to make acid before the stomach contents are removed. You will need to avoid eating or drinking for 6 hours before the test. During the test you may feel mild discomfort or a gagging feeling as the tube is passed through your nose or mouth, and down into your esophagus.

You may need this test for the following reasons:

• If you have severe indigestion that cannot be relieved with treatment, which may be due to lack of acid production by the stomach.

• To check if anti-ulcer medications are working.

• To check if contents are being regurgitated back up from the small intestines which is not normal.

• To see if there is bile in the stomach, which indicates contents are backing up from the small intestine (duodenum). This may be normal but can indicate digestive problems and poor intestinal motility. It may also happen after part of the stomach is removed with surgery.

• To test for the cause of peptic (stomach and/or duodenal) ulcers.

The stomach acid test is very safe as you are fully conscious. There is a slight risk of the tube being placed through the windpipe and into the lungs instead of through the esophagus and into the stomach.

Results of stomach acid test:

Normal results:

The volume of the stomach fluid is 20 to 100 mL

The acid level (pH) is acidic (1.5 to 3.5).

Gastric Motility Studies
(Test to measure rate at which stomach empties)

A gastric emptying study is a test that uses radioactive chemicals to measure the speed that food empties from the stomach and enters the small intestine. Gastric emptying studies are done in patients who are having symptoms that may be due to too slow or too rapid emptying of the stomach. The symptoms of slow emptying include reflux, nausea, vomiting, and abdominal fullness after eating. The symptoms of rapid emptying are diarrhea, weakness, or dizziness after eating.

For a gastric emptying study, the patient eats a special meal containing a small amount of radioactive material. A scanner over the patient's stomach monitors the amount of radioactivity in the stomach for several hours after the test meal is eaten. As the radioactive food empties from the stomach, the amount of radioactivity in the stomach decreases. The rate at which the radioactivity leaves the stomach demonstrates the rate at which food is emptying from the stomach

Hiatus Hernia

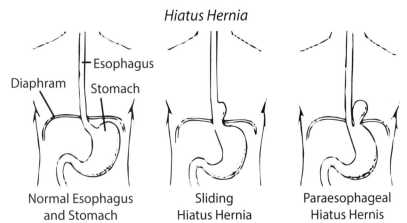

Normal Esophagus and Stomach

Sliding Hiatus Hernia

Paraesophageal Hiatus Hernis

Glossary - *Recipes*

Arrowroot - Is similar to cornstarch and is also used as a thickening agent. It can be used to thicken soups and gravies, instead of flour, and in baking biscuits and cakes. Is gluten free.

Banana Leaf - Young banana leaves can be used for cooking and wrapping food. They can be bought and trimmed to size. Always cut the mid rib away. Most Asian shops and grocers will stock them. I have even seen them in some supermarkets. They will keep in the freezer for several months.

Carob Flour - Made from the carob bean, may be a substitute whenever chocolate or cocoa is used.

Coconut - when buying desiccated or shredded coconut, always sniff the packet; it will smell rancid if it is off, even through the plastic.

Coconut Milk - is the white milky liquid that is extracted from the flesh, not the clear milk inside the coconut. It can be bought in cans from the supermarket or Asian stores.

Cold Pressed Oil - all your oils i.e. olive, almond, walnut, coconut, avocado, flaxseed, etc. should be stored in the dark, either under the sink or in a cupboard, as this extends the shelf life and stops them from going rancid. If buying oil in large quantities, store the main container, and use a funnel to pour the oil into a dark or green glass bottle for daily use.

Couscous - is made from semolina (it is not gluten free) and can be used in sweet and savory dishes. It is an alternative to rice and pasta.

Dry Roast - To place either nuts, seeds, spices and some flours in a heavy saucepan, without any liquid, and constantly moved over a high flame to release the flavor, aroma and natural oils. Makes a delicious seasoning.

Fish Sauce - A dark colored sauce used mainly in Asian cooking. It is made from anchovies marinated in vinegar and water and is quite healthy.

Flour - There are many types of flour, that can be used for cooking. Mung bean, carob, chestnut, oat, buckwheat, barley, rice, arrowroot, amaranth, quinoa, spelt, chickpea (Besan), hemp seed flour, corn, rye, soy, lentil, potato and wheat to name a few. To make the flour self raising, add 1 teaspoon of baking powder.

Some ideas of whole wheat substitution might be

1 cup of whole wheat flour (plain) = 1/2 cup soy flour + 1/2 cup arrowroot or any one of the following

3/4 cup rice flour

1 cup corn flour

1+1/4 cups barley flour

3/4 cup potato flour

1+1/3 cups oat flour

1+1/3 cups soy flour

Julienne - The name given to food strips, (firm foods are easier to work with), ie. carrots, chillies, ginger, celery, capsicums etc, cut into thin, long strips.

Marinate - To soak foods in a liquid mixture, to either flavor, soften (tenderize) or preserve.

Miso - A paste made from fermented beans, usually soya. Other varieties include, barley and rice. Sweet or savory. It can be used to make a quick nutritious probiotic soup, stock, or spread on bread.

Mushrooms - There are many delicious varieties, such as shiitake, field (wild), porcini and button to name a few. When exploring Asian green grocers, keep an eye out for exotic, fresh and dried varieties. Experiment with a combination of mushrooms for the various recipes. When using dried mushrooms, always soak in water for approximately 30 minutes before cooking. Mushrooms can be a source of selenium and are good for the immune system.

Purée - To make foods into a smooth consistency using a blender, food processor or masher.

Rice Noodles - Made from rice and water. Available in different thicknesses, from a flat wide noodle to thin vermicelli. The thin variety can be soaked in hot water for 20 minutes. Can be bought fresh or dried.

Sambal - A hot and spicy relish, usually made from crushed chillies and vinegar.

Seaweeds - are really sea vegetables. They are very high in iodine and calcium; thus they are good for the bones and immune system. Can be used in soups, stir fries and other dishes. Some tasty varieties are, Hijiki, Nori, Kombu, Agar Agar, Arame and Wakame.

Agar Agar - Is made from sea vegetables and used to set jellies and mousses etc. It can be used exactly like gelatin. It needs to be cooked or simmered for several minutes in water before setting.

Arame - A thin (thread), black sea vegetable. Great in salads and rice.

Hijiki - A nutty, salty sea vegetable. Before adding to soups and stir fries, soak for around 10 minutes. Kombu - Is a large, flat, dark green sea vegetable. It is mainly used for stocks and soups. Good with beans and other vegetables.

Nori - Comes in dark brown or green sheets or ribbons. It is a sea vegetable and is generally used to make sushi. It can be bought toasted or plain. When using nori to make sushi, it needs to be toasted slightly. To toast - quickly pass nori over a gas flame on each side, till crispy. Store in an airtight container in a dark place.

Wakame - A long, thin sea vegetable. Good for stocks and soups. It can be used dry, if baked - crumbled on top of salads and vegetable dishes.

Shoyu - is very similar to soy sauce, but is not chemically processed. It is a little sweeter and slightly more salty than tamari.

Soy Sauce - Available as either dark (a little sweeter) or light (saltier), and is made from fermented soya beans and wheat. Look for naturally brewed soy sauces that do not contain chemical additives.

Tamari - is similar to soy and shoyu but is less salty and has no wheat. Is very tasty and can be used whenever soy sauce is needed, as a wheat/gluten free substitute. Is a by-product of the miso making process.

Tempeh - is made mainly from fermented soybeans, but can be made from other beans and nuts. It has a very nutty flavor and is more firm and compact than tofu. Can be used interchangeably with tofu.

Tahini - Is a paste made from toasted/untoasted sesame seeds. It can be either hulled (white) or unhulled (brownish). It is very high in calcium and good for the bones. Great for spreads, dressings, sauces etc.

Tofu - Is made from soybeans. It is low in calories and fat. Great for those who are wanting to lose weight. It can be used in soups, desserts and stir fry dishes. It can be substituted for most chicken dishes and many of the seafood dishes in this book.

Umeboshi - A pickled plum which has a salty/sour taste. It is used for salad dressings, with vegetables and is great with rice.

Wok - is an Asian saucepan. It has sloping sides and is very handy. When the ingredients at the bottom are cooked, they can be moved up the side and the uncooked ingredients moved down. It can be used to steam, stir fry and also deep fry any foods.

Glossary- *Medical*

Amino Acids- a group of organic compounds identified by the presence of both an amino group (NH2) and a carboxyl group (COOH). They are the building blocks for protein and are essential to life. Although around 80 amino acids are found in nature, only 22 are needed for human metabolism. The ones that cannot be produced by the body, and must be supplied by food, are called essential amino acids. The essential amino acids are histidine, isoleucine, leucine, lysine, methionine, cysteine, phenylalanine, tyrosine, threonine, tryptophan, and valine. The non-essential amino acids (which the body can manufacture itself), are alanine, aspartic acid, arginine, citrulline, glutamic acid, glycine, hydroxyglutamic acid, hydroxyproline, norleucine, proline and serine. Arginine can be essential in certain states or age groups because the body cannot make it fast enough to supply the demand.

Anus - the outlet of the rectum through which feces are expelled. It is found between the buttocks.

Auto-antibodies - proteins formed by the immune system (known as immunoglobulins), which attack the tissues of the body.

Autoimmune Disease - diseases where the immune system is unable to distinguish its own tissues from foreign substances. The immune system produces antibodies against normal body tissues, which results in inflammation and injury.

Bacteria - microorganisms that can be shaped as a sphere, a rod or a spiral. They grow in colonies, usually composed of the descendants of a single cell. All animals and humans carry bacteria on and inside their bodies, and some have the potential to cause serious diseases. Many bacteria produce toxins. Bacteria are the principle agents of decay and putrefaction of organic substances.

Carcinogenic - capable of causing cancer.

Cat Scan (CAT) - computerized X Ray, looking at the body in slices.

Chlorophyll - the green pigment found in plants, which absorbs sunlight. This pigment has health benefits when consumed in green colored foods.

Chronic - long drawn out illness, with slow progression; the opposite of acute illness.

Colonic Irrigation - washing or flushing out the colon with high enemas, consisting of large amounts of fluid.

Colitis - inflammation of the colon.

Damaged Fats - dietary fats whose chemical structure has been changed from its natural state by oxidation induced by light, hydrogen, heat and oxygen or chemical manufacturing processes.

Dairy Products - cow's milk and its products such as butter, cheese, cream, yogurt, ice cream and chocolate.

Detoxification - reduction of the toxic properties of a poisonous substance through a series of chemical reactions. This occurs principally in the liver cells.

Digestion - the process of breaking food down into smaller particles, so it can be absorbed from the intestines into the blood stream and utilized by the body.

Dysfunction - impaired, inadequate or abnormal function of an organ, or part of the body.

Enzymes – these are complex protein substances produced by living cells. Enzymes act as catalysts and induce chemical changes in other substances without being changed themselves. Enzymes are present in digestive juices, where they act upon food substances, breaking them down into smaller simpler substances. They are present in every cell, especially in the liver and enable the liver cells to breakdown drugs and toxins. They can speed up chemical reactions and processes involved in both breaking down substances or building new substances.

Esophagus - that portion of the digestive tract that extends from the back of the throat to the stomach.

Essential Fatty Acids (EFAs) - unsaturated fatty acids that cannot be manufactured by the body and must be obtained in the diet. EFAs are essential to good health. These include linolenic acid, arachidonic acid and linoleic acid

Fats - substances made up of one molecule of glycerol combined with three fatty acids. The fats found in body tissues are made up of fatty acids, especially oleic acid, palmitic acid and stearic acid. See also lipids.

Fat-soluble - substances dissolving in fatty tissues or oily liquids only.

Fungi - a species of plant-like organisms that includes yeasts and molds. Fungi grow as single cells as in yeast, or as multi-cellular filamentous colonies, as in molds and mushrooms. Many forms are pathogenic to animals and plants.

Gallbladder - pear shaped sac on under surface of right lobe of liver. The gallbladder stores bile from the liver until it is discharged through the bile duct into the intestines during a meal.

Gastroenterologist - a physician with postgraduate training and qualification in the diagnosis and treatment of diseases affecting the digestive system.

Genetic - pertaining to the genes (found on the chromosomes) of the organism or species. Concerned with hereditary characteristics and reproduction.

Genetic Engineering - the alteration, manufacture or repair of genetic material by man-made technology

Genome - the complete set of genes in an organism. Also the total genetic content in one set of chromosomes. The human genome is made up of approximately 35,000 genes. The fruit fly has 13,300 genes, the roundworm - 18,300 genes and mustard weed has 25,700 genes. More than 98% of human DNA is identical to chimpanzee DNA.

Genotype - the genetic makeup of an individual. The combination of alleles located on chromosomes that determines a specific characteristic or trait.

Glandular System - the network of glands that manufacture hormones. Also known as the endocrine system. Gluten - a protein found in certain grains, especially wheat, rye, barley and oats.

Hemorrhoid - a mass of dilated veins occurring around the anus or rectum.

Hepatitis - inflammation of the liver.

Hiatus hernia - a protrusion of a portion of the stomach up through the diaphragm into the chest cavity.

Hydrogenation - a chemical process used to turn liquid oils into solid form. This is achieved by passing hydrogen atoms through the oil under high pressure. Hydrogenation impairs the nutritional value of the oil and produces distorted fatty acid molecules that do not occur in nature.

Hypoglycaemia - abnormally low level of sugar (glucose) in the blood.

Immune System - a system that exists in the body to identify and eliminate foreign and harmful substances or microorganisms that have invaded the body. It consists of specialized cells that produce antibodies and/or ingest these foreign things. The lymphatic system, bone marrow, thymus gland, spleen and liver, all play vital roles in the efficient functioning of the immune system.

Immunoglobulins - proteins manufactured by the cells of the immune system that attack or neutralize foreign substances or microorganisms. They are also known as antibodies.

Infection - invasion of body tissues by disease causing microorganisms, such as viruses, protozoa, parasites, bacteria or fungi.

Inflammation - redness, heat, swelling, and sometimes pain, occurring in tissues injured by various means such as infection, burning, excess acidity, trauma or toxins.

Jaundice - yellow discoloration of the skin and mucous membranes caused by a build up in the body of bile pigments.

Lactase - an enzyme that exists in the intestinal lining and is required to digest the sugar found in milk (lactose).

Lactose Intolerance - an inability of the body to metabolize the sugar found in milk (lactose), which is due to deficiency of the enzyme lactase. Symptoms include diarrhea, abdominal cramps, bloating and gas.

Lipase - the enzyme produced by the pancreas that breaks down fats into smaller absorbable substances. Lipids - fatty substances which are insoluble in water, and dissolve in fat solvents such as chloroform and alcohol. Lipids include esters of fatty acids and glycerol, phospholipids and cholesterol.

Lipoproteins - molecules consisting of proteins combined with lipids such as cholesterol, phospholipids and triglycerides. Blood fats do not circulate in an unbound or free state, but are chemically bound to proteins, which enables them to be transported safely.

Lymphocytes - white blood cells forming part of the immune system.

Malnutrition - deficiency of nutrients essential to health

Metastases - deposits of cancer cells that are growing in sites of the body distant to their source of origin. Microorganisms - minute living bodies, not perceived by the naked eye, eg. a bacterium or parasite.

Metabolism - the physical and energy transformations that exist within living cells.

Mitochondria - the energy factories inside every cell.

Mucus - the viscous (glue-like) secretions of the mucous membranes composed of mucin, salts and body cells.

Oxidation - the chemical process in which oxygen reacts with another substance, causing it to change. These changes usually result in some damage or deterioration (similar to rust). Oxidation often liberates free radicals, which cause further damage.

Pancreas - a gland situated behind the stomach. It lies in a horizontal position with its head attached to the duodenum and its tail reaching to the spleen. It produces digestive enzymes which enter the duodenum, and the hormones insulin and glucagon which control glucose metabolism.

Pancreatitis - inflammation of the pancreas.

Parasite - an organism that lives within, upon, or at the expense of another organism, known as the host, without contributing to survival of the host.

Pathogenic - capable of producing disease.

Pernicious Anemia - a form of anemia, caused by deficiency of vitamin B12. This deficiency arises because the small intestine is unable to absorb vitamin B12 from food or vitamin B supplements. Thus vitamin B12 injections must be given.

Phytonutrients - nutritional substances beneficial to health found in plants.

Protease - an enzyme produced by the pancreas to breakdown food proteins into smaller amino acids so they can be easily absorbed from the gut.

Tumor - swelling or enlargement. A spontaneous new growth of tissue, forming an abnormal mass.

Villi - the finger like projections covering the surface of the inner lining of the intestines that are designed to increase the absorptive area of the intestinal tract.

Virus - a minute organism not visible with ordinary light microscopy. It is a parasite dependent upon nutrients inside cells for its metabolic and reproductive needs. Viruses can be seen by using an electron microscope and consist of a strand of either DNA or RNA (but not both) surrounded by a protein covering.

Water-soluble - substances dissolving in watery tissues/liquids and not in fat..

Bibliography - *References*

Fujimura K E, et al. Role of the gut microbiota in defining human health. Expert Rev Anti Infect Ther. 2010 Apr;8(4):435-54. doi: 10.1586/eri.10.14.

R A Rastall Bacteria in the gut: Friends and foes and how to alter the balance. The Journal of Nutrition August 1, 2004 vol. 134 no. 8 2022S-2026S

Patrice D Cani and Nathalie M Delzenne Interplay between obesity and associated metabolic disorders: new insights into the gut microbiota. Current Opinion in Pharmacology 2009, 9:737–743

Rogler G. Prebiotics and probiotics in ulcerative colitis: where do we stand? Digestion. 2011;84(2):126-7. Epub 2011 Apr 15

Sartor RB. Efficacy of probiotics for the management of inflammatory bowel disease. Gastroenterol Hepatol (N Y). 2011 Sep;7(9):606-8

Barbara G, Zecchi L, Barbaro R, et al. Mucosal permeability and immune activation as potential therapeutic targets of probiotics in irritable bowel syndrome. J Clin Gastroenterol. Oct 2012;46 Suppl:S52-55

Bouhnik Y, Alain S, Attar A, et al. Bacterial populations contaminating the upper gut in patients with small intestinal bacterial overgrowth syndrome. Am J Gastroenterol. May 1999;94(5):1327-1331

Mi-Ran Ki et al. Lactobacillus paraplantarum isolated from kimchi inhibits Helicobacter pylori growth and adherence to gastric epithelial cells. J Med Food. 2010 Jun;13(3):629-34

(Corley 2010) Life Extension, Gastro-esophageal Reflux Disease. www.lef.org

Benjamin J et al. Glutamine and Whey Protein Improve Intestinal Permeability and Morphology in Patients with Crohn's Disease: A Randomized Controlled Trial. Dig Dis Sci. 2011 Oct 26

Den Hond E, Hiele M, et al. Effect of long-term oral glutamine supplements on small intestinal permeability in patients with Crohn's disease. JPEN J Parenter Enteral Nutr 1999;23(1):7-11

Sido B, Seel C, Hochlehnert A, et al. Low intestinal glutamine level and low glutaminase activity in Crohn's disease: a rational for glutamine supplementation? Dig Dis Sci 2006;51(12):2170-9

Kuroki F, Matsumoto T, et al. Selenium is depleted in Crohn's disease on enteral nutrition. Dig Dis. 2003;21(3):266-70

Margaret Rayman, Dietary Selenium: time to act, British Medical Journal Vol. 314, 387, 8th Feb. 1997

Brozmanova J. Selenium and cancer: from prevention to treatment. Klin Onkol. 2011; 24(3):171-9.

Naithani R. Organoselenium compounds in cancer chemoprevention. Mini Rev Med Chem. 2008 Jun;8 (7):657-68.

Clark LC, et al. Effects of selenium supplementation for cancer prevention in patients with carcinoma of the skin. A randomized controlled trial. Nutritional Prevention of Cancer Study Group. JAMA. 1996 Dec 25; 276(24):1957-63.

Ganther HE. Selenium metabolism, selenoproteins and mechanisms of cancer prevention: complexities with thioredoxin reductase. Carcinogenesis. 1999 Sep;20(9):1657-66.

Rayman MP. Selenium in cancer prevention: a review of the evidence and mechanism of action. Proc Nutr Soc. 2005 Nov;64(4):527-42.

Fleet JC. Dietary selenium repletion may reduce cancer incidence in people at high risk who live in areas with low soil selenium. Nutr Rev. 1997 Jul;55(7):277-9.

Peters U, Takata Y. Selenium and the prevention of prostate and colorectal cancer. Mol Nutr

Food Res. 2008 Nov;52(11):1261-72.

Yoshizawa K, et al. Study of pre-diagnostic selenium level in toenails and the risk of advanced prostate cancer. J Natl Cancer Inst. 1998 Aug 19;90 (16):1219-24.

Ghadirian P, et al. A case-control study of toenail selenium and cancer of the breast, colon, and prostate. Cancer Detect Prev. 2000;24(4):305-13.

Willett WC, et al. Pre-diagnostic serum selenium and risk of cancer. Lancet. 1983 Jul 16; 2 (8342):130-4.

Salonen JT, et al. Association between serum selenium and the risk of cancer. Am J Epidemiol. 1984 Sep;120 (3):342-9.

Glattre E, et al. Prediagnostic serum selenium in a case-control study of thyroid cancer. Int J Epidemiol. 1989 Mar;18 (1):45-9.

Mark SD, Qiao YL, et al. Prospective study of serum selenium levels and incident esophageal and gastric cancers. J Natl Cancer Inst. 2000 Nov 1;92(21):1753-63.

Van den Brandt PA, et al. A prospective cohort study on selenium status and the risk of lung cancer. Cancer Res. 1993 Oct 15;53 (20):4860-5.

Helzlsouer KJ, Comstock GW, Morris JS. Selenium, lycopene, alpha-tocopherol, beta-carotene, retinol, and subsequent bladder cancer. Cancer Res. 1989 Nov 1;49(21):6144-8.

El-Bayoumy K. The negative results of the SELECT study do not necessarily discredit the selenium-cancer prevention hypothesis. Nutr Cancer. 2009;61(3):285-6.

Marshall JR, et al. Methyl Selenocysteine: single-dose pharmacokinetics in men. Cancer Prev Res (Phila). 2011 Aug 16.

Fleming J, Ghose A, Harrison PR. Molecular mechanisms of cancer prevention by selenium compounds. Nutr Cancer. 2001;40 (1):42-9.

Sinha R, El-Bayoumy K. Apoptosis is a critical cellular event in cancer chemoprevention and chemotherapy by selenium compounds. Curr Cancer Drug Targets. 2004 Feb;4 (1):13-28.

Fang MZ, Zhang X, Zarbl H. Methylselenocysteine resets the rhythmic expression of circadian and growth-regulatory genes disrupted by nitrosomethylurea in vivo. Cancer Prev Res (Phila). 2010 May;3(5):640-52.

Bhattacharya A. Methylselenocysteine: a promising antiangiogenic agent for overcoming drug delivery barriers in solid malignancies for therapeutic synergy with anticancer drugs. Expert Opin Drug Deliv. 2011 Jun;8(6):749-63.

Bhattacharya A, et al. Magnetic resonance and fluorescence-protein imaging of the anti-angiogenic and anti-tumor efficacy of selenium in an orthotopic model of human colon cancer. Anticancer Res. 2011 Feb;31(2):387-93.

Langmead L et al. Anti-inflammatory effects of aloe vera gel in human colorectal mucosa in vitro. Aliment Pharmacol Ther. 2004b Mar 1;19(5):521-7

Koutroubakis IE, Malliaraki N, et al. Decreased total and corrected antioxidant capacity in patients with inflammatory bowel disease. Dig Dis Sci. 2004 Sep;49(9):1433-7.

Langmead L et al. Randomized, double-blind, placebo-controlled trial of oral aloe vera gel for active ulcerative colitis. Aliment Pharmacol Ther. 2004a Apr 1;19(7):739-47

Vallejo F, et al, "Phenolic compounds in edible parts of broccoli inflorescences after domestic cooking" Kidmose U and Kaack K. Acta Agriculturae Scandinavica B 1999:49(2):110-117

Song K and Milner J A. "The influence of heating on the anticancer properties of garlic," Journal of Nutrition 2001;131(3S):1054S-57S

Watanabe F, Takenaka S, Abe K, et al, J. Agric. Food Chem. Feb 26 1998;46(4):1433-1436

George D F, Bilek M M, and McKenzie D R. "Non-thermal effects in the microwave induced unfolding of proteins observed by chaperone binding,"

Quan R (et al) "Effects of microwave radiation on anti-infective factors in human milk," Pediatrics 89(4 part I):667-669.

Bai Y, Xu MJ, Yang X, et al. A systematic review on intrapyloric botulinum toxin injection for gastroparesis. Digestion. 2010;81(1):27–34.

Kim EK et al. Fermented kimchi reduces body weight and improves metabolic parameters in overweight and obese patients. Nutr Res. 2011 Jun;31(6):436-43. http://pmid.us/21745625.

Won TJ et al. Therapeutic potential of Lactobacillus plantarum CJLP133 for house-dust mite-induced dermatitis in NC/Nga mice. Cell Immunol. 2012 May-Jun;277(1-2):49-57. http://pmid.us/22726349.

Won TJ et al. Oral administration of Lactobacillus strains from Kimchi inhibits atopic dermatitis in NC/Nga mice. J Appl Microbiol. 2011 May;110(5):1195-202. http://pmid.us/21338447.

Hong HJ et al. Differential suppression of heat-killed lactobacilli isolated from kimchi, a Korean traditional food, on airway hyper-responsiveness in mice. J Clin Immunol. 2010 May;30(3):449-58. http://pmid.us/20204477.

Park KY et al. Kimchi and an active component, beta-sitosterol, reduce oncogenic H-Ras(v12)-induced DNA synthesis. J Med Food. 2003 Fall;6(3):151-6. http://pmid.us/14585179.

Kim HJ et al. dimethoxyphenyl)propionic acid, an active principle of kimchi, inhibits development of atherosclerosis in rabbits. J Agric Food Chem. 2007 Dec 12;55(25):10486-92. http://pmid.us/18004805.

Kim YS et al. Growth inhibitory effects of kimchi (Korean traditional fermented vegetable product) against Bacillus cereus, Listeria monocytogenes, and Staphylococcus aureus. J Food Prot. 2008 Feb;71(2):325-32. http://pmid.us/18326182.

Sheo HJ, Seo YS. The antibacterial action of Chinese cabbage kimchi juice on Staphylococcus aureus, Salmonella enteritidis, Vibrio parahaemolyticus and Enterobacter cloacae. J Korean Soc Food Sci Nutr 2003, 32:1351-1356. Hat tip Rafael Borneo, http://dietasaludperfecta.blogspot.com.ar/2013/03/kimchi-un-superalimento.html.

Zhang YW et al. Effects of dietary factors and the NAT2 acetylator status on gastric cancer in Koreans. Int J Cancer. 2009 Jul 1;125(1):139-45. http://pmid.us/19350634.

Nan HM et al. Kimchi and soybean pastes are risk factors of gastric cancer. World J Gastroenterol. 2005 Jun 7;11(21):3175-81. http://pmid.us/15929164.

Lee SA et al. Effect of diet and Helicobacter pylori infection to the risk of early gastric cancer. J Epidemiol. 2003 May;13(3):162-8. http://pmid.us/12749604.

Lee SA et al. Effect of diet and Helicobacter pylori infection to the risk of early gastric cancer. J Epidemiol. 2003 May;13(3):162-8. http://pmid.us/12749604.

Seel DJ et al. N-nitroso compounds in two nitrosated food products in southwest Korea. Food Chem Toxicol. 1994 Dec;32(12):1117-23. http://pmid.us/7813983.

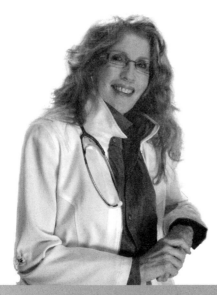

Other Titles by Sandra Cabot MD

**Order by calling my
Health Advisory Service on
+1 623 334 3232
or order from the website**

www.liverdoctor.com

Alzheimer's - What you must know to protect your brain and improve your memory

With no current cure for Alzheimer's, this book is essential reading for those who don't want to leave the fate of their brain to chance. Your brain is fragile and vulnerable to the epidemic of dementia. Contains Dr Cabot's 4 point program to prevent and slow down the progress of dementia. Also includes tips on caring for loved ones.

Bird Flu - Your Personal Survival Guide

Your immune system is your greatest asset and protects you against infections, cancer and inflammation. Learn how to have a strong immune system. Provides effective help for fighting all viruses. This book is vital for anyone with chronic infections and indeed for every man and woman in the street.

The Body Shaping Diet

You can change your body shape! The Body Shaping Diet is a reliable and scientific way of eating for your particular body shape. It provides foods to suit you - your body shape, metabolism and hormonal type - enabling you to shed excess weight from where you want to.

Boost Your Energy

Finetune your body and mind with natural anti-ageing hormones and immune boosting nutrients. Strategies and information on how to overcome Chronic Fatigue Syndrome. Includes a 14 day energy diet and exercise plan.

Breast Cancer Prevention Guide

Breast cancer is the most feared disease for the majority of women - yet most feel powerless over their ability to prevent it. Many women believe breast cancer is a result of bad genes and bad luck. The truth is: only five to ten percent of breast cancer cases are genetic. New research has shown that nutritional and environmental factors appear to be the biggest culprit in the alarming increase in breast cancer rates. Learn the key factors to keeping your breasts healthy in the Breast Cancer Prevention Guide.

I Can't Lose Weight and I Don't Know Why

Have you tried all the fad diets, exercised your heart out and still wonder why you can't lose weight? This is the book for you. Understanding successful weight control is like solving a jigsaw puzzle. Each piece interacts with every other, and without an understanding of how they all fit together you cannot complete the big picture. A piece can be as simple as a deficiency of iodine or as complex as hormone imbalance, thyroid resistance, food addiction, body inflammation and many other causes. Learn what each piece of the puzzle is and what to do about it.

Cholesterol: The Real Truth

Are the drugs you're taking making you sick? Cholesterol is NOT the real cause of heart disease! Discover powerful foods to lower your bad cholesterol and a natural program to reduce heart attack and stroke. Learn about the dangers of cholesterol lowering drugs.

Diabetes Type 2: You Can Reverse It Naturally

The conventional dietary advice given to diabetics can actually make the disease worse. Diabetics should not follow low fat diets because all carbohydrates are digested into sugar, and raise blood sugar levels. Why manage diabetes with diet and medication when you can actually reverse it? This new book contains a two week meal plan and more than 40 recipes suitable for Type 2 diabetics to lose weight and lower blood sugar levels.

Endometriosis Your Best Chance To Cure It -e-Book

This **e-book** explains in simple terms everything you need to know about endometriosis and outlines the steps that need to be taken to cure it long term. Many women think there is no hope of really curing this serious disease or falling pregnant once diagnosed with this condition. With the information in this book, which you can implement in your own life, there is an excellent chance, not only of a positive outcome, but a complete cure.

Available from on-line bookstores like Amazon, GooglePlay and iTunes.

Fatty Liver: You Can Reverse It

Fatty liver disease is the most common type of liver disease seen in the world today. Dr. Cabot tells us that reversing fatty liver disease is not only an effective method of losing weight, but can also greatly reduce the most common diseases of today - namely diabetes, heart disease and cancer. Dr. Thomas Eanelli describes his battle with his own liver disease and food addiction in the section of the book, Confessions of a Fat Man. His fight for survival takes him on a journey - both physical and mental - to find his inner power and physical health.

Help For Depression and Anxiety

In this book, Dr Cabot provides you with practical help to overcome emotional illness, stress, anxiety and unhappiness. It is important to understand the brain's chemistry so that we can achieve the chemistry of happiness and realise our full potential! A practical plan that you can tailormake for yourself to gain more control over your emotions and state of mind so that you can become the best you can be.

Increase Your Sex Drive

Dr Sandra Cabot sees thousands of women who ask for help with their sex life - they want to improve it for themselves and they want to improve their relationship with their lover. Not every woman likes to talk about it and often believes there is nothing she can do to get her mojo back. No matter what age you are, it is possible to have a sex life and it can be a really wonderful one!

Infertility: The Hidden Causes

Infertility is not a disease; rather it is a symptom of an underlying health problem. Once these health problems are identified and remedied, in most cases fertility will be restored. In this well researched book, Dr Sandra Cabot and naturopath Margaret Jasinska explore the many hidden causes of infertility which are often easily overcome. A healthy body is a fertile body.

Low Carb Cocktail Party

Most people like to enjoy an alcoholic beverage occasionally or for a special event. Miss Madeleine Hotcakes has designed these fabulous recipes from her years of experience as a well known bartender in London and New York. Madeleine's cocktail recipes are different because they are not only delicious, they are all natural and low in carbohydrates. They are made with natural whole fruits and not fruit concentrates, thus they are high in antioxidants.

Hormones - Don't Let Them Ruin Your Life

Hormones are the most powerful chemicals in your body. They have the power to be physically and emotionally shattering or they can make you feel wonderfully alive. Provides solutions for endometriosis, polycystic ovarian syndrome, pituitary problems, contraceptive dilemmas, acne, hair loss and facial hair.

Hormone Replacement - The Real Truth

Dr Cabot provides the latest information on menopause and discusses natural bio identical HRT and how it can change your life. Strategies for anti-ageing, mood disorders and the pain of Fibromyalgia. Includes phytoestrogen rich recipes to reduce your risk of cancer and osteoporosis.

How Not To Kill Your Husband

Balancing your hormones can save your marriage, as well as your husband's life. Chances are that you are angry, frustrated, tired and just over it. That's your perspective and it's real and probably justified – hey, who wants to be a perfect superwoman and mum and wife at the same time? The expectations on women these days to be everything to everybody whilst under the influence of hormonal upheaval can be enough to see you reach breaking point. Buy this book to help yourself or your daughters or perhaps to save your marriage.

The Liver Cleansing Diet - Over 3 million copies sold

The award winning book that opened the eyes of the world to the importance of this forgotten organ. The ground breaking concepts in this book made Dr Cabot a household name. Published in many different languages, it has sold over 3 million copies. The eight week liver cleansing diet and the vital principles for a healthy liver will enable you to "love your liver and live longer"! Despite its vocal critics, those who followed this award winning diet, not only managed to lose weight but rediscovered their health.

Magnesium the Miracle Mineral

MAGNESIUM can be LIFE SAVING, as it is known to reduce the risk of sudden death from cardiac catastrophes – this is particularly important for men under stress. Dr Cabot's book looks at many different and common health problems, that can surprisingly be relieved, or at the very least, significantly helped, by simple and safe supplementation with magnesium. Magnesium is a mineral that can make a huge difference to your health and yet many people, even in the developed world, have inadequate magnesium levels in their body.

Raw Juices Can Save Your Life

Dr Cabot says, "I have seen juicing work miracles in many of my patients who were stuck on the merry-go-round of drug therapy and told they had incurable diseases." This book provides a complete A-Z guide of juicing recipes for various health conditions. Raw juicing can restore health, even in those with seemingly hopeless and chronic conditions. (Also available in Mandarin)

Save Your Gallbladder Naturally and what to do if you've already lost it

A comprehensive step by step plan for dissolving gallstones and improving gallbladder function. A book to help everyone affected by disease of the gallbladder or bile ducts. If you are having gallbladder problems, whether you have already lost it or not, this book tells you what to do. Gallbladder disease can be painful and frightening, which explains why many people are rushed off to surgery to have their gallbladder removed. These decisions are complex and serious and thus it takes an expert in liver and gallbladder problems, like Dr Sandra Cabot, to help you make sense of it. Some people still have the same pain after surgery, some people never feel well after having their gallbladder removed. Thankfully, Dr Cabot has written this book to help you and your doctor make the best decisions. In most cases there are safe natural alternatives.

Tired of Not Sleeping?

Discover holistic solutions for nearly 70 things that could be stopping you from getting a good night's sleep! There is always a cause for insomnia which can be treated. Learn about the correct use of anti depressant drugs, foods to help your brain relax, herbal sleeping remedies and melatonin.
This book provides you with practical strategies for 68 things that stop you sleeping, such as: Depression, anxiety, sleep apnea, snoring, hot flushes, muscle cramps, itching skin, painful joints and muscles and much more.
Sleep is your safety valve - you must get a good night's sleep!

The Ultimate Detox

A two week deep cleaning diet; the quickest and safest way to restore your health. This program works on all the detoxification systems in the body and will leave your aura shining! Dietary plans are free of gluten and dairy and are suitable for vegans. Do you suffer with toxic overload?

This two week deep cleansing diet will get your aura shining!

This book gives you life-saving strategies to

• Rid your body of dangerous toxins
• Repair your bowel
• Fight micro-organisms with natural antibiotics

Want to Lose Weight But Hooked On Food?

During Dr Cabot's years of research into emotional overeating, she found one of the major problems that kept people from achieving their goal weight was their toxic belief system. No matter what they did – what diet they pursued or how much they exercised – nothing happened. Their limited belief system held them back, or their achievements were short-lived. This limited belief system is the reason behind the negative selftalk, which leads to negative feelings, which lead to emotional overeating.

Your Thyroid Problems Solved

Is your thyroid gland making you sick?

Try Dr Cabot's thyroid check list:

• Are you always tired?
• Do you struggle to lose weight?
• Are you depressed?
• Do you suffer with fluid retention and puffiness?
• Do you often feel cold?
• Is your memory & concentration poor?
• Are your bowels sluggish?
• Is your hair thinning, dull & lifeless?
• Are your muscles weak & sluggish?

If you have several of these problems –

You could be suffering with a thyroid gland problem. Thyroid disease is far more common than originally thought and thousands of people may be undiagnosed. This well researched and scientific book gives you holistic guidance to the management of thyroid conditions.